Orange is the New Pink

Orange is the New Pink

My Battle with Triple-Negative Breast Cancer

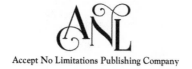

Accept No Limitations Publishing Company

Orange is the New Pink
My Battle With Triple-Negative Breast Cancer
Marquita Bass

ISBN: 978-1-948018-67-8, Softcover
ISBN: 978-1-948018-68-5, eBook

Disclaimers: Although the author and publisher have made every effort to ensure that the information in this book was correct at press time, the author and publisher do not assume and hereby disclaim any liability to any party for any loss, damage, or disruption caused by errors or omissions, whether such errors or omissions result from negligence, accident, or any other cause. This book is not intended to provide any medical advice. The reader should consult a physician in matters relating to health and particularly with respect to any symptoms that may require diagnosis or medical attention.

ANL

Accept No Limitations Publishing Company

Dedication

This book is dedicated to the following women who have died from triple-negative breast cancer.

• Valerie Lyles – You were my beautiful, stylish, and kind neighbor for more than 15 years. I miss you.

• Aunt Addie "Felicia" Barnes – Auntie, you were my beautiful role model. Thank you for taking my secrets to the grave. I am still grieving your death, seven years later.

• Mary Dehaye – Your friendship, life, and encouragement propelled me to write this book. I miss talking to you on the phone. We didn't make it to the gun range where we were going to pretend we were shooting cancer cells. My heart is sad.

• Maleikka H. Williams – Lovely Lady, you were too young to die at age 36. Your husband and two wonderful daughters miss you. Your girls are thriving.

This book is also dedicated to my friends who are currently dealing with breast cancer. Thank you for allowing me to be a part of your journeys. I appreciate the encouragement and support you gave me while I wrote my book. I pray for you often. I love you.

This book is also dedicated to my family and friends who are breast cancer survivors. Your strength, courage, and determination give me hope. Thank You, God!

Acknowledgements

First of all, I would like to thank the Living God, who has given me strength and perseverance to see this project to its completion. "Thanks be to God through Jesus Christ our Lord!" (Romans 7:25).

To my wonderful parents, the beloved Clifford Ricks, Jr., and Helen Ricks, thank you for being intelligent and exemplary role models and teachers. Thank you for raising me to be a person of faith, courage, and dignity.

To my son, Christopher, you were my reason for fighting for my life during my cancer journey. Thank you for playing your saxophone, keyboard, or drums when I felt sad and scared, and insisting that I listen to you. The music was soothing and therapeutic, although our neighbors may feel differently. I love you, *Scooter Boodle.*

To Diletha Waldon, thank you for helping me with the book title. I could not have come up with a great title without your help. You are amazing.

To Diane Loupe, thank you for helping me with the book subtitle and the foundational book edits. You challenged me to search *my soul* and to speak *my truth,* uncensored.

Thank you to everyone who showed up for me before and after my surgery.

A special acknowledgment goes to Veena N. Rao, Ph.D., professor at the Morehouse School of Medicine and co-director of the Cancer Biology Program in Grady's OB/GYN Department. Thank you, Dr. Rao, for taking time out of your busy schedule to give me a tour of your cancer lab. As you showed me the various instruments and the repositories where tumor cells are stored, I felt inspired and excited about cancer research. You are brilliant, sympathetic, kind, and fundamentally a good person. Thank you for your research efforts and commitment to finding targeted treatments for triple-negative breast cancer. Thank you for your time, information, and support.

Dr. Rao is the first woman to receive the Mario Toppo Distinguished Scientist title. She has dedicated her research to understanding the BRCA1 gene and its mutations. Her goal is to improve medical treatment of African-American women with breast cancer. Dr. Rao's research has led to the development of a patented technology, when combined with BRCA1 DNA-based testing, promises to revolutionize early detection of hereditary triple-negative breast cancers, foster development of novel targeted therapies, and save countless lives.

Contents

Introduction

If you have breasts or love a woman with breasts, this book is for you. Although males also get breast cancer, I have limited the scope of this book to breast cancer in females. Having breasts is the *Number 1* risk factor for getting breast cancer.

The goals of this book are: to share information about breast cancer by walking you through my journey, to encourage women (especially young women) to understand their breast cancer risk factors and to manage them, and to increase awareness of triple-negative breast cancer (TNBC). My objective as I wrote was DMSU: Don't Make Stuff Up. Thus, I have included a lot of references, especially in Chapter 9, where I focus on cancer research.

I am an extremely private person, so the thought of writing a book about a personal life tragedy is out of character for me. Therefore, I had to summon courage after I made a promise to my late friend, Mary DeHaye. As Mary was transitioning, she asked me to tell my story because "too many women are dying from triple-negative breast cancer, and there needs to be more public awareness. Also, TNBC patients need the same type of treatment options that are available for other types of breast cancers." Yes, breast cancer is not one disease. Mary also asked me to share my story about how I ended up with bright orange hands after I finished cancer treatment.

TNBC is an aggressive breast cancer with a poor prognosis for approximately 30 to 40% of patients (this percentage could be different, depending on the study). More disturbing, there are four or six subtypes (depending on the study). Yet, the different subtypes are not addressed by oncologists in a clinical setting. However, research and clinical trials are ongoing and promising. I pray for the day that TNBC is not treated as one disease, as several studies have shown that the subtypes are molecularly different, and thus respond differently to therapeutic agents.

Triple-negative breast cancer showed up in my life like a meteor out of nowhere. The foundation of my life was shattered; however, I have emerged as a victor seven years after my diagnosis. Each day, I thank God for the present day. Cancer is an insidious disease, and I don't know what tomorrow will bring.

Everyone's breast cancer experience is different and unique due to our distinct physiology. I am not a medical doctor or a research scientist, and I would never recommend or give my opinion on treatment options. What a woman decides to do with her body is personal and a decision that should be made between her and a medical doctor.

In order to protect the innocent, I have changed the names of the doctors and other personnel who treated me. However, I didn't change the names of friends, family, and researchers.

CHAPTER 1

"Bad news isn't wine. It doesn't improve with age."
~ COLIN POWELL

It's a Cancer

"MS. BASS, ARE YOU still on the line? Ms. Bass, are you still on the line?" Dr. Mullins repeated.

Finally, I heard her voice and replied, "Sorry. Yes, I am."

Then she said, "I have made an appointment for you to come into the office today to speak to the surgeon. Can you make it? I thought you would want to come in as soon as possible."

I replied, "Yes I will be there, and thank you for getting me in today. Goodbye."

On Tuesday, May 22, 2012, I was anxiously waiting for Dr. Mullins to call me with my breast cancer biopsy results. When she called around 2 p.m., my heart started beating rapidly. I asked the doctor if I could put her on hold while I walked to a private area. As I rushed down three flights of stairs to the mother's room in the building where I worked, I almost slipped and fell. Out of breath, I sat down in a chair, took the doctor off hold, and nervously asked, "Do you have the biopsy results?"

I'll never forget what the doctor replied, "Ms. Bass, It's a C A N C E R."

I almost slumped over in the chair and hit the floor from surprise. I couldn't believe the doctor had given me a cancer diagnosis over the phone. But I was sure it was because she had picked up on my anxiety during the breast biopsy, so I was relieved she didn't make me wait for the results. Thank you, Dr. Mullins.

My next thoughts after I heard the horrifying word "cancer" were, "What about Christopher? He needs both of his parents." Christopher is my only child, and he was in the eighth grade. He was my entire world and my reason for living, my lifeline. I felt a deep sense of despair. As those thoughts rushed through my head, the line was silent. That's why Dr. Mullins asked me if I was still on the line.

It was beyond my imagination to think that I might miss Christopher's high school and college graduations. I could not imagine missing him grow into a mature adult. The cancer diagnosis was earth-shattering. It was as if I were outdoors in the midst of a tornado—smack in the eye of a tornado, and I didn't have any control over my body movements. The winds of my emotions were blowing so hard; I was forced to search for something to hold onto. There I was, 48 years old, and I didn't want to die.

It was a very hectic day at work when the doctor called. I am a project manager who is ambitious, a high achiever, detail-oriented, and conscientious. That day, I was working on a major high-visibility project that was very stressful. Earlier in the day, as I was meeting with team members, updating the project schedule, and negotiating with outside consultants, my stomach was in painful knots. The discomfort made me feel anxious and nauseated.

Nevertheless, I was able to appear as though I was okay with no worries in the world, other than being a good project manager. No one knew what was going on with me. I didn't even tell my coworker and friend, Terri, with whom I shared my life experiences daily.

THE EVENTS THAT LED up to the May 22 diagnosis had started on May 14 with a routine mammogram. I had gone to a breast care facility in North Atlanta and didn't expect anything out of the ordinary. That feeling changed as soon as the nurse practitioner showed me the tumor with the jagged edge on my mammogram film. I felt alarmed. It was as if the tumor was looking back at me with an evil smile, saying, "Hi there! I am cancerous." The nurse practitioner explained that the ultrasound that followed the mammogram had confirmed the radiologist's concerns that the tumor looked equivocal, which meant it could be cancerous—but maybe was not. To allay my fears, she also said it was small and most likely, not cancer. The scheduler made an appointment for me to return four days later for a breast biopsy.

During this time, I was living with my niece, Laquisha. My son was living with his father fulltime instead of every other week, which was our usual schedule as co-parents. Christopher and I had had to rush out of our home in the middle of the night after I asked my ex-husband to sprinkle mothballs in the attic to get rid of squirrels. The pungent smell of mothballs made our home uninhabitable.

ON MAY 17, 2012, the night before my breast biopsy, Laquisha and I watched *Grey's Anatomy*. In the episode, the medical team was involved in a plane crash. I had never watched the show before, so I didn't understand why the episode involved a plane crash instead of hospital scenes. My niece gave me the rundown on what was happening. The show seemed good, but I had other things on my mind. I started Googling on my laptop as though I were working on a research paper.

With an irritated look, Laquisha asked, "Why are you on the computer instead of focusing on the show? Do you ever just watch television, Auntie Quita?"

I laughed and replied, "No, you know your auntie is a multi-tasker." We both burst out laughing.

Next, I said in a matter-of-fact tone, "Tomorrow, sweetie,

the doctor is going to do a biopsy on a tumor in my right breast. It looked suspicious on a recent mammogram and ultrasound. I have breast cancer, so I am on the internet researching what I am going to do."

Laquisha jumped up from the couch, paused the show, and looked at me like I had two heads or was on hard drugs. "How do you know it is cancer?" she demanded. "You are stressing out for no reason! Watch the show Auntie!"

I explained that the tumor appeared to have a jagged edge, so I felt like it was cancerous based on research I had previously done.

According to an article published on the National Center for Biotechnology Information (NCBI) website, the most significant features that indicate whether a mass is benign or malignant are its shape and margins. The shape can be round, oval, lobular, or irregular. Circumscribed oval and round masses are usually benign. An irregular shape suggests a greater likelihood of malignancy.[1]

Then I told her, "I am going to have a bilateral mastectomy. I am chopping off both of these puppies."

She was floored. "Auntie Quita, you are over the top as usual. You don't have breast cancer!"

"I love my breasts. I am a size 6, and I love to wear my 32G Panache bras. I pray to God that I don't have cancer. Do you want to hear about some of the sexual tricks your auntie can do with these puppies?" I said.

Before Laquisha could respond, I lifted my T-shirt and said, "Look at me: my breasts look like two perfectly shaped large balloons on the outside. However, the balloons are fibrocystic with breast calcifications on the inside. Now, I have a tumor with a jagged edge."

My niece looked at my breasts and said, "Whoa! Wow! They are huge. I didn't know your breasts were that large. How do you hide them?"

I was silent. Laquisha returned to watching *Grey's Anatomy*, and I returned to my Google search:

- How do you look after a mastectomy?
- Is there a lot of pain after a mastectomy?
- Are breast implants safe?
- How long does it take to recover after a mastectomy?
- What is the survival rate for breast cancer?

BY THE TIME I arrived for my biopsy at the breast care facility on May 18, I was struggling to remain calm. In my mind, I had already started working on my treatment plan. As a project manager, I know how to take charge, handle tough situations, and deal with bad news. Still, I was very nervous and anxious. Dr. Mullins and the ultrasound technician greeted me with smiles. They asked me personal questions about my life and my family in an attempt to keep me comfortable.

"What do you have planned for the weekend?" the doctor asked. I could feel her warmth and care. The doctor explained that most small tumors are benign. It didn't matter; I still could not focus on what she was saying. I was in the *Twilight Zone*. I would have preferred to be in a *Feel-Good Zone* from drinking Patron shots. Where was the tequila?

During the biopsy, I was awake. My body was stiff and tense on the exam table; it was like I was in a coma. As Dr. Mullins explained the procedure and wiped my breast with orange-colored antiseptic swabs, I blurted out, "If it is cancer, I am going to chop off both breasts. I have already researched what I am going to do."

The doctor seemed amazed by what I was saying. Her body language said: "I can't believe what this patient said." However, she maintained her composure and professional disposition as she began the procedure.

At that moment, I was horrified by the terrifying journey

that might be in store for me. At the same time, I wanted to appear to be in control because I had a plan. Or, was I trying to be strong because that was how I had been taught to behave when life throws you a curveball? Throughout my life, my mom always told me, "Only the strong survive." Also, I could hear my father's voice saying, "Baby girl, handle your business." I was trying to be strong and handle my business, but it was tough.

My brain felt like it was on steroids, and all kinds of thoughts raced through my head. Can a doctor tell if a tumor is cancerous after she looks at the tissue sample during a biopsy? Does a cancerous tumor sample have a distinct smell, color, or texture? Will the biopsy cause cancer to spread?

After the doctor placed the tissue sample in a container and placed a bandage on my small incision, she said, "I will see you later." I thought, "Was that a Freudian slip? Does the tumor specimen look like it is cancerous, which is why she is saying she will see me later?"

Dr. Mullins' last words were, "I will call you by Tuesday next week with the results. Enjoy your weekend."

As I walked quickly to my car, I went from thinking in my head to talking out loud.

I shouted, "I don't want to talk to that doctor or any doctor ever again. I definitely don't want to see her again.

"I don't want to deal with breast cancer.

"I don't want to chop off my girls.

"I don't want to go to work and deal with the project I am working on.

"Forget about this! I didn't sign up for this experience. This is unadulterated bull crap."

Suddenly, I felt embarrassed. I stopped and looked around the parking lot to see if anyone was listening or watching me. I spotted a young woman with a concerned look on her face standing near her car. She was watching me walk and talk. I felt crazy—it was an insane experience. As I got into my car, I wondered what she was thinking. "It's official," I thought, "I am crazy."

ACCORDING TO THE AMERICAN Cancer Society, breast cancer is the most common cancer in U.S. women, and the second leading cause of death. It is estimated that 252,710 women in the U.S. will be diagnosed with invasive (cancer cells have moved to surrounding tissue) breast cancer and 63,410 will be diagnosed with in situ (cancer cells are contained in milk ducts) breast cancer in 2018, and 40,610 women will succumb to this disease during this time.[2] Do the statistics bother anyone besides me? Furthermore, breast cancer is **NOT** one disease. *This is an important fact that women need to understand.*

Doctors use many terms to describe breast cancer tumor characteristics: cancer type, histology, molecular make-up, tumor marker receptor, tumor grade, the list goes on. Therefore, I have developed the *4 Ts of Breast Cancer* to make it easy to understand the most common breast cancer diagnosis.

Aunt Quita's Understanding of Breast Cancer

"TO" is for Tumor Origination: Where did your cancer originate or where does it reside?

A. Ductal –Milk ducts carry milk from glands. If the tumor is contained in a milk duct, it's referred to as non-invasive or DCIS. If the tumor has spread to the surrounding tissue, it is referred to as invasive. According to Breastcancer.org, about 80% of all breast cancers are invasive ductal carcinomas or (IDC).[3]

B. Lobular – A lobule is a gland that makes milk. If abnormal cells are present in the lobules, a person is at higher risk of getting breast cancer in the future. If the abnormal cells become malignant and break through the lobule walls, this is invasive lobular carcinoma (ILC).[4]

<u>C. Inflammatory Breast Cancer (IBC)</u> – This is an extremely rare form of breast cancer that is fast growing. According to the American Cancer Society, about 1% of all breast cancer cases in the United States are inflammatory breast cancers. Inflammatory breast cancer usually starts with the reddening and swelling of the breast instead of a distinct lump.[5]

Unfortunately, I have a good friend who went through treatment for invasive lobular carcinoma. One evening, we sat in a restaurant for more than three hours discussing breast cancer. I think my heart skipped a beat when I saw the tormented and confused look on her face, as she asked, "How could I have gotten mammograms for the last 10 years and end up with Stage 3 Invasive Lobular Breast Cancer?" I was speechless and felt sad.

Later, I rushed home and spent hours looking for an answer. ILC is the second most common type: 10% of breast cancers.[6] As it turns out, invasive lobular breast cancer is not generally a solid tumor. In my friend's case, it presented as malignant speckles across one of her breasts that almost reached her chest wall. According to breastcancer.org, invasive lobular carcinomas tend to be more difficult to see on mammograms than invasive ductal carcinomas, because, instead of forming a lump, the cancer cells more typically spread to the surrounding connective tissue (stroma) in a line formation.[7]

My friend's cancer didn't show up on either a mammogram or an ultrasound screening. If her radiologists had not noticed unusual breast density during a mammogram compared to previous images, the cancer might have gone undetected. Moreover, "studies and a meta-analysis of those studies suggest that the relative risk of invasive lobular, compared to invasive ductal cancer, is particularly affected by combined hormone replacement therapy (HRT) in postmenopausal women, with an approximate doubling of the risk of invasive lobular breast cancer in current users."[8]

My friend was almost 50 and taking birth controls pills when she was diagnosed. Her cancer treatments included surgery and radiation therapy. Because female hormones stimulated the growth of the ILC, my friend is taking an aromatase inhibitor drug to reduce the amount of estrogen in her body. As far as lifestyle changes, I have never seen anyone jump on the healthy living bandwagon as quickly as she did. Immediately, my friend eliminated sugar and dairy from her diet and switched to a plant-based diet. I feel confident that she will remain cancer free.

Please listen carefully: I am not suggesting that birth control pills caused my friend's cancer. However, birth control pills and hormone replacement therapy are synthetic hormone medications: the same drugs wearing different suits. Interestingly, the medical experts who wrote *The breast cancer epidemic: 10 facts*, stated: "Hormones, both in the form of combined hormone replacement therapy and combined oral contraceptives increase the risk of breast cancer.[9] Also, several peer-reviewed articles state that *a woman's lifetime exposure to estrogen and progesterone are a risk factor for developing breast cancer.*

In her book, *Breasts: The Owner's Manual*, Dr. Kristi Funk, states, "estrogen levels, growth factors, new blood vessel formation (angiogenesis), inflammation, and immune system function are factors that affects a tumor's microenvironment— the fluids and cells that bathe, support and fuels cancer....or seek and destroy them." Dr. Funk is a renowned breast cancer surgeon. In a girlfriend style of writing, she does an excellent job explaining the biology of breasts and breast cancer risk factors. My hope is that her book will encourage women to think about their breast health and risk factors before they pink. Pink is the color associated with breast cancer, so women should consider learning about their individual breast cancer risk factors in order to possibly reduce their chances of dealing with the disease. Please refer to Appendix A for a list of breast cancer risk factors.

Is it unreasonable to think that there could be some correlation or even causation between my friend's invasive lobular carcinoma and being on birth controls pills at the time of her diagnosis? I don't know; it's something to consider.

Another more important million-dollar question, why aren't women who have taken female hormones either as birth control pills or hormone replacement therapy routinely screened with MRIs because ILC may not show up on mammograms and ultrasounds, and 10% of breast cancers originate in the lobules? The cost of getting the appropriate breast cancer screening based on your particular risk factors for breast cancer is "PRICELESS."

Another friend, Jae, is currently thriving and living with Inflammatory Breast Cancer. As I previously mentioned, IBC is rare. Ten years before her diagnosis, Jae was diagnosed with DCIS breast cancer, the tumor was contained in a milk duct. Her treatment for DCIS included a lumpectomy and high-dose radiation therapy. In addition, she took Tamoxifen for 5 years. Later, Jae was horrified when she was diagnosed with Stage 3 Inflammatory Breast Cancer. She said, "I didn't want to leave my husband alone to raise our kids. My family needed me." The second time around, Jae had a bilateral mastectomy and took chemotherapy. Although the average life expectancy for IBC is 57 months, Jae has passed that checkpoint. My amazing friend is claiming victory, daily. She told me, "I am not going anywhere, I am very stubborn, and I can't leave my family." I am inspired by Jae's determination and drive to beat the odds. She is living proof that cancer statistics do not apply to an individual. Jae's cancer treatments, lifestyle changes, and raw determination are keeping her alive.

For additional information on less common types of breasts cancers, please refer to Appendix B.

Now that we understand where the nightmare tumor may originate in the breasts, we need to understand the tumor biology/molecular structure.

"TB" is for Tumor Biology: What is the molecular make-up of your tumor?

When a pathologist examines a breast tumor, she looks for three receptors on the tumor to determine the molecular biology of the cancer, or tumor marker receptors. **Receptors** are like antennas attached to the tumor that respond to signals from either estrogen or progesterone. The pathologist also examines the level of a protein called human epidermal growth factor receptor 2 (HER2). This protein promotes the growth of breast cancer. The following table outlines the four major molecular/biology structures of breast cancer, according to the American Cancer Society Breast Cancer Facts and Figures 2017-2018.

Breast Cancer Molecular Structures

	Estrogen/ Progesterone	HER2	Responses	Prognosis
Hormone positive, Luminal A (71%)	Positive	Negative	Tumor grows in response to female hormones and not to an overexpression of HER2.	Better outlook in the short-term, but these cancers can sometimes come back many years after treatments.[10,11]
Hormone Positive, Luminal B (12%)	Positive	Positive	Tumor grows in response to female hormones and to an overexpression of HER2.	Tend to be higher grade and are associated with poorer survival than Luminal A cancers.[11]
Triple-Negative (12%)	Negative	Negative	Tumor is not fueled by either female hormones or an overexpression of HER2.	A poorer short-term prognosis than other subtypes, in part because there are currently no targeted therapies for these tumors.[12]
HER2-Enriched (5%)	Negative	Positive	Tumor is not fueled by female hormones but there is an overexpression of HER2.	The recent widespread use of targeted therapies for HER2+ cancers has improved outcomes for these patients.[11]

"TS" is for Tumor Size.

The size of the tumor is measured at its widest point, usually in millimeters (mm). Although patients with smaller tumors may have a better outcome, size doesn't give the whole picture and is just one part of the overall equation. A small tumor can be fast growing while a larger tumor may grow slowly, or it could be the other way around. *Early cancer detection* is important. You want to catch the cancer before it spreads to the lymph nodes and other areas in the body.

"TG" is for Tumor Grade: How fast are the cells growing?

Cancer cells are given a grade according to how different they are from normal breast cells and how quickly they are growing, according to breastcancer.org/uk.

There are three grades of breast cancer:

1. Grade 1 – looks most like normal breast cells and is usually slow growing.
2. Grade 2 – looks less like normal breast cells and is growing faster.
3. Grade 3 – looks different than normal breast cells and is usually fast growing.

AFTER I FINISHED TALKING to the doctor, I placed my phone on a table, sat for about 30 minutes, and stared at the blue wall in front of me. Several thoughts zoomed through my head as though I were reading from a teleprompter.

- I try to eat a plant-based diet.
- I only drink alcohol a few times a year.
- I am at my ideal BMI, and I exercise.
- I use crystal deodorant to avoid aluminum.
- I have never smoked tobacco products.
- I have stayed away from oral contraceptives, except for 3 months to treat acne.

Because I didn't think I was at risk for breast cancer, I was in absolute disbelief and shock. I knew that I had a few relatives with breast cancer, but I had consciously tried to live a lifestyle that would not lead to a breast cancer diagnosis. I had avoided foods, products, and medications that would disrupt my endocrine system. So, I stood up and started pacing around in circles in the small mother's room and asked myself, "Why me? What have I done to deserve a breast cancer diagnosis?"

A reality check is a way to bring a person back to the truth and facts of her circumstances. The reality was: my doctors had been monitoring a suspicious area in my right breast for four years. Unfortunately, the suspicious area had presented as a cancerous tumor. Did the reason that this was happening matter? It didn't matter at the time; I needed to focus on the next steps.

Immediately, I grabbed my phone and called my coworker Sandra who is a breast cancer survivor. She and I had had extensive conversations about breast cancer. Unfortunately, she and my Aunt Addie were diagnosed with breast cancer at nearly the same time, a few years earlier. Sandra's treatments for hormone-positive cancer included surgery and chemotherapy. I had watched my coworker fight her disease with the fortitude of a gladiator. She was determined to beat cancer, so she was brave and declared victory from the beginning. Sandra made lifestyle changes after her diagnosis that included stress reduction and improving her diet.

Surprisingly, I was calm as Sandra and I talked about my diagnosis. She assured me that I would be okay, then she warned me that the journey was going to be hard. I could not get the word "hard" out of my mind. In the past, I was used to overcoming adversity and hard situations. But the words "hard" and "cancer" coupled together terrified me. Sandra could sense my fear, so she said emphatically, "Marquita, whatever you do, don't have a pity party. You have to think positive and maintain hope." She was right! I have noticed that women who try to remain positive and who have hope tend to have more favorable outcomes.

After Sandra left, I called my Aunt Addie who was dying from metastatic triple-negative breast cancer disease. Cancer that has spread to other parts of the body is called metastatic cancer.[13] Without asking my aunt how she was doing, I stuttered and struggled to say, "It's cancer; I have breast cancer."

She fired off questions at me like a prosecutor cross-examining a murder suspect. Her voice sounded like she was in a fight for my life as well as for her own. Addie was born to be an interrogator. When her nieces went to her for advice, we knew Addie was going to ask a lot of questions and give us a solution. She knew how to dissect an issue to get to the root cause of a problem. If we asked for advice about a new man, Addie asked: "What is his name? Does he have a job? Where did you meet him? Why do you like him? Has he ever been married? Is he married? How do you know he is telling the truth?" Aunt Addie was our rock. She was hilarious, borderline nosy, and a loving pain. However, we never hesitated to reach out to our aunt when we needed advice.

"What do you mean you have breast cancer?" Addie asked with exasperation. "Did you have a breast biopsy? Where are you? When did you find out? Who is your doctor? Are you okay? Do I need to come to you?"

As I struggled to respond, I started crying uncontrollably. Surprisingly, no one knocked on the door or called security even though I was wailing like a toddler throwing a temper tantrum. Sitting in that small room at work, I had a sudden urge to throw my cell phone at the wall. Then, I realized—oh my goodness—my aunt has metastatic triple-negative breast cancer! Why am I freaking out over an initial breast cancer diagnosis? But I could not stop crying, blowing my nose, and freaking out. That was the *only* time during my cancer journey that I cried when another person could hear me.

Addie's voice was soft and calm as she said, "Breathe, Quita, and try to calm down." I was shocked by what she said next. "Make sure you *only* use a breast surgeon and not a general surgeon for whatever surgery you may decide to have."

I thought, "Why is she talking about who I should use as a surgeon? I don't know anything about the biology of my cancer. I don't have any facts. I don't know the type, size, or stage of my cancer."

The line was very quiet. Addie sensed my confusion, so she told me that she had used her general surgeon for her bilateral mastectomy, and the results were less than favorable. "I am in no way suggesting that a general surgeon can't deliver good breast cancer surgery results," she said. "I am simply sharing my experience."

I stayed in the mother's room until it was time for me to leave work and head to my appointment to meet with the breast surgeon.

"Acting is magical. Change your look and your attitude,
and you can be anyone."

~ ALICIA WITT

Let the Curtain Go Up

AS I LEFT WORK on that Tuesday, I struggled to pull myself together. All I could think about were the words, "It's a cancer." I could not get the doctor's voice out of my mind. As I headed to the breast cancer center, I cried, and the words, "It's a cancer," played over and over in my head.

My eyes were red and puffy; I was distraught. At one point, I almost crashed into a car in front of me. The near collision startled me so much that I shouted, "Get it together, Marquita." I had to whip cancer's butt, so I made a conscious decision to focus on driving. I put on my full Armor of God and let the show begin.

There I was, the leading lady in a play for which I had not auditioned, in a role I did not want.

CHRISTOPHER WAS GOING TO be at the breast center on the day I visited the surgeon because his father had to pick him up from school. I didn't want to alarm my son. We are very close, and he is very in tune with my actions and feelings, paying attention to my every move. Whenever he sensed my stress, he asked, "What's wrong? Why are you looking like that? Do you ever sit down and do nothing, Mom?"

Laquisha, Jerome, and Christopher met me in the parking lot. No one uttered a word, not even "hi." I asked them to follow me; we glanced at each other and started walking into the doctor's office. I wondered what my child was thinking. After school, Christopher typically attended band practice, a tutorial, or rehearsed for the school play. Surprisingly, he showed no indication that he thought something might be wrong until we were seated in the waiting room.

I signed in at the registration desk and sat down between Jerome and Christopher. Then I asked my son if anything happened at school that he wanted to discuss. He was at an age where it was like pulling teeth to get him to answer questions about his school day. Christopher would usually say nothing more than, "School was good." On the other hand, if I asked my son a question about his music lessons or marching band rehearsal, he was a motor mouth. I was excited that he was enthusiastic about music.

That day, to my surprise, Christopher responded in full sentences when I asked him about his day. I could see his lips moving, but I could only hear background sounds from the television in the waiting area. I didn't hear my son's words until he asked, "What is wrong with you, Mom?"

Fighting back tears, I replied, "I will be okay, Son."

The nurse came out and asked me to follow her, saying, "I will return after your exam to retrieve your family members." It was perfect timing—I didn't want to talk to my son any longer. And I definitely couldn't cry in front of him. I leaned over and whispered in Jerome's ear, "You are welcome to come back when the nurse returns for the family, but please leave Christopher in the waiting area."

He nodded his head, "Okay."

As I waited for the breast surgeon to enter the examination room, I sat on the exam table upright and as stiff as a statue. I held my gown together and clasped my arms tightly across my chest. I needed to protect the girls. I thought, "Is this for real? What about Christopher? I don't want to die before he graduates from high school."

Then I had a déjà vu moment and started thinking about my mom's death from pancreatic cancer when I was a junior in college. She had been 49; I was now 48. It felt like I had already been a character in a similar story. Thinking back, I am surprised the doctor didn't walk into the room and find me passed out on the floor. I was terrified. But I *acted* like I was okay.

A very attractive breast surgeon who appeared to be in her forties walked in and introduced herself as Dr. Stallone. "I am sorry to meet you under these circumstances. You are the second patient today with a breast cancer diagnosis. May I please conduct a breast examination before we discuss your biopsy results?" In my mind, I wanted to reply, "No, and if you come near me, I am going to jump off this exam table and run for my life."

Instead, I said, "Yes, you may."

It is interesting how throughout my cancer journey, one response would immediately pop up in my head, while the words out of my mouth were different.

The doctor talked as she examined me, but the only words I heard were, "I can't feel the tumor, so the scans are the only way we would have found this. I am glad you stayed on top of your health and breast screenings."

If it had not been for two amazing doctors in my life who payed close attention to my health, I would have missed or ignored important health red flags that showed up two years before I was diagnosed in 2012. Red flag number one was chronic hives that appeared out of nowhere all over my body one night. My boyfriend at the time rushed over to my house with ointments and Benadryl because I was hysterical.

To treat the hives, I consulted Dr. Strause, an African-American dermatologist in Buckhead, an upscale neighborhood within the city limits of Atlanta. She could have prescribed a strong ointment and antihistamines and sent me on my merry way. Because Dr. Strause is a thorough and caring physician, she ordered antibody blood work that revealed I had Hashimoto's disease. It is an autoimmune disorder caused by the production of abnormal antibodies. Autoimmune disease is where the immune system attacks normal mechanisms in the body, which could be a sign of other conditions. According to an article in The Lancet, *Breast Cancer in Patients With Hashimoto's Thyroiditis,* "patients with Hashimoto's thyroiditis are one high-risk population for breast cancer."[1]

After that diagnosis, I attempted to take better care of myself by adding more iodine to my diet, and I tried to reduce the stress in my life. I didn't know what was driving the illness. A year later, I ended up in Dr. Strause's office with shingles, which is a viral infection that causes painful rashes. Thankfully, I only had a mild case. I was trying to eat healthy meals and exercise more, so my immune system may have kept the shingles at bay.

Again, Dr. Strause could have simply prescribed an anti-viral medication for my shingles and stopped there. However, she insisted that I follow-up with my primary care doctor because my immune system was working overtime for some reason. She said, "Your overtaxed immune system could be why the dormant chickenpox virus in your lower spine is active again." I was consumed with raising my son, work, and in an emotionally challenging relationship, so I didn't follow up with my primary care doctor. However, I heard what Dr. Strause was saying, so I continued to try to exercise more and eat healthy meals.

Since my diagnosis, I have met several breast cancer patients who told me they had either shingles or some type of skin condition prior to their diagnosis. I am not suggesting that every woman who is diagnosed with an autoimmune disease or rash will end up with breast cancer. There may not be a cause-and-effect relationship; but, pay attention to your body and try to work with your doctor to address disease symptoms and probable causes. If your doctor only focuses on horses, she may miss the zebras.

BEFORE MY BREAST CANCER diagnosis, Dr. Brenner, my excellent gynecologist of 25 years, asked me during a routine visit if I was staying on top of my breast screenings. I mumbled something about needing to make an appointment. Looking somewhat grim, my gynecologist urged me to make an appointment as soon as possible. "Your last mammogram shows breast calcifications. I want you to remain diligent about your breast health," she said. At that moment, I felt special and grateful that she was reading the reports from the breast center. Again, I felt fortunate to have a team of dedicated and caring doctors.

A good doctor can be the difference between life and death. The word "good' is subjective and may take on different meanings for each of us.

For me, a good doctor:
• Attempts to get to know her patients.
• Is focused on the patient's total health.
• Reads patient's medical reports from other doctors.
• Actively listens to her patients.
• Stays abreast of medical research.
• Typically finds the zebra.

My life was chaotic at that time, so I know I would not have scheduled my mammogram when I did if my gynecologist had not insisted that I be vigilant about my breast health. I was managing one of the most difficult projects I had ever worked on in my life, suffering with the emotional pain from a breakup with a man I loved from the core of my heart, grieving the death of my brother who died seven months earlier from lung cancer, worrying about Aunt Addie's metastatic breast cancer, managing the care of my disabled Veteran sister, and staying on top of

Christopher's school work and music lessons. I am surprised, I survived. It was a tumultuous time in my life.

With so much going on, I was overwhelmed and trying to manage my stress. Therefore, making doctor appointments was not a priority, which was a huge mistake. A lot of women make their kids, spouses, significant others, work, and other family members their priority while neglecting themselves. In my rush to make sure everyone else I loved was taken care of, I almost made a fatal omission.

AFTER THE SURGEON FINISHED examining me, she told me to get dressed, and the nurse would escort me to another room. While the surgeon and I waited for my family to join us, I looked up and saw Laquisha, Jerome, and—guess who—my son, walk through the door. My son was 13 and in middle school. He didn't know why he was at the doctor's office with me instead of following his typical after-school routine.

Remember, I had asked my ex-husband, Jerome, to leave our son in the waiting room, and he had agreed. He had obviously forgotten what he had agreed to. I almost blew a gasket when I saw my child. But I quickly noticed the concern and sadness on my ex-husband's face. He seemed disoriented and confused. Jerome saw a scale and told Christopher, "Look, Son, here is a scale. I wonder how much I weigh."

Immediately, I jumped up and walked over to Jerome, touched him on the arm and whispered in his ear, "Please take Christopher back to the waiting room and stay with him until we return."

With a look of relief on his face, Jerome turned around and followed my directions like an obedient child. Jerome's sister told me, a few years later, that he had been devastated by my cancer diagnosis. He was afraid that I was going to die, which explains why he appeared to be discombobulated at the doctor's office.

After Jerome and Christopher left, Laquisha took notes and recorded every word the breast surgeon said. The doctor took her time to explain my results, and she dumbed down the information to keep it simple.

The breast surgeon told me that:

- I had a 12 mm tumor, which is considered small.
- The tumor is located at about 12 o'clock in my right breast.
- She would know the biology of my breast cancer in two days. It could be hormone-positive, HER2, or Triple-Negative. The information would be in a second pathology report.
- The more aggressive the cancer, the more aggressive the treatment.
- Survival rates for breast cancer have improved.
- First, there is local treatment, which could be a lumpectomy followed by radiation or a mastectomy.
- Second, there is distant treatment, which may include chemotherapy with possible use of other drugs like Tamoxifen.
- I needed to schedule an MRI to look at both breasts in more detail to make sure we didn't miss anything.

Even though I had walked into her office in a fog, I was able to focus on every single word Dr. Stallone said. After she finished talking, I responded without pausing to take a breath. For some bizarre reason, I felt like, "I got this." I went through the motions and *acted* like the strong person I thought I had to be. I spoke as though I were reading from a script and reporting the evening news from the anchor's chair.

"My aunt has metastatic triple-negative breast cancer, which I am sure you know is a very aggressive form of breast cancer.

"So, I am going to chop off both breasts. I am NOT going to get

breast reconstruction because my aunt had something called expanders after her reconstruction. It has been a nightmare for her. She got an infection in her skin, and the skin would not heal or stretch. My aunt traveled back and forth to some doctor in Athens, Georgia, to get something filled. And, her breasts still aren't right, and my aunt is dying. I would prefer to not have breasts and have a flat chest instead of having to deal with what my aunt is going through.

"Also, my cousin had a lumpectomy last year, and she had to go back. The doctor didn't get all the cancer the first time. The margins or something was not good. No lumpectomy and radiation for me—the thought of still having mammograms after this experience would stress me out.

"Also, my neighbor died from metastatic triple-negative breast cancer. How do I schedule the MRI?"

With a sympathetic look on her face, Dr. Stallone replied, "Call the office in the morning to schedule the MRI; and I can support a bilateral mastectomy [i.e., removing both breasts] because your mammogram films show that you have very busy breasts." By very busy, I assumed she was referring to my fibrocystic breasts and breast calcifications that had started showing up on my mammograms prior to my diagnosis.

Dr. Stallone added, "I understand your concern about the expanders. The plastic surgeon may be able to skip the expanders if you have enough good skin after surgery to cover your implants. You may want to consider how your clothes will look; you may want to swim. More importantly, you should consider the psychological impact of having a flat chest if you skip breast reconstruction. You are young and would have a lot of years to live without breasts."

There was silence. Laquisha looked up from the notebook to see my reaction.

I thought, "Are you kidding me? I don't care if I never swim or see another beach in my life. I am sure there are pads or something that I can wear in my bra if I don't have reconstruction surgery. What about a breast prosthesis?"

The only thing that mattered to me at that time was my son. I had to live for him. And I didn't want to leave him like my mom had left me when she died at 49. But I didn't say any of this out loud. Finally, I thanked the surgeon for staying after hours to meet with me, and the consultation was over.

Dr. Stallone stopped by her assistant's office to find business cards for a couple of plastic surgeons after she walked us out. She encouraged me to see a plastic surgeon to discuss breast reconstruction before I made a final decision. Dr. Stallone was phenomenal: she was smart, caring, sincere, and patient. She answered all of my questions, and she answered some questions multiple times, without hesitation. She was a class act.

Laquisha and I rejoined Jerome and Christopher in the waiting area. As we walked to our cars, no one uttered a word. As I drove back to my niece's house, Aunt Addie called to tell me that I had an appointment at Emory Winship Cancer Institute where she was receiving treatment. My aunt wanted me to get a second opinion, so she and her husband had arranged for me to meet immediately with a second breast surgeon.

The emotional storm I was in raged on, but I didn't let anyone see my fear.

CHAPTER 3

"One's philosophy is not best expressed in words; it is expressed in the choices one makes ... and the choices we make are ultimately our responsibility."
~ ELEANOR ROOSEVELT

Making Tough Decisions

AFTER A BREAST CANCER diagnosis, you feel like your house has been destroyed by a natural disaster, and now you have to make quick decisions to rebuild your life. Before I made any decisions about my breast cancer diagnosis, I scheduled a physical with my primary care physician. The goal was to ensure that I was aware of any other potential health conditions that could influence my decisions related to breast surgery and treatments. I had an awesome and compassionate primary care physician, Dr. Bates, who saw me the next day after I contacted her office. She was my rock throughout my entire journey, and she remained my physician until she closed her private practice in Lithonia, Georgia.

During the exam, she recognized that I was a total wreck and suffering from major anxiety, so she gave me the following Scripture to read.

Philippians 4:6 NIV: *Do not be anxious about anything, but in every situation, by prayer and petition, with thanksgiving, present your requests to God.*

If it had not been for Dr. Bates, I think I would have suffered a nervous breakdown as I prepared for surgery. She asked me how much time I needed at work to wrap up things so she could put me under her care until my surgery. Otherwise, I would have worked up until the day of surgery. Boy, I really needed the time off because I could barely function. Furthermore, my anxiety level was high and unmanageable. Also, I had to run back and forth to doctors, have additional tests, and make tough decisions.

To complicate matters, I was still dealing with squirrels in my attic and the pungent smell of mothballs. I ended up replacing all the insulation to remove the mothballs so I could return home. It was a nightmare that added to the stress of dealing with a cancer diagnosis. The pain associated with a cancer diagnosis and working with the insulation contractor was difficult, so my ex-husband stepped in to make sure the contractors removed all the mothballs and properly replaced the insulation. I was thankful for Jerome's help.

Decision #1 – Who will be my breast surgeon?

On Friday, May 25, 2012, Laquisha and I headed to the Winship Cancer Institute at Emory University for a second opinion. Dr. Styles walked into the exam room and greeted me by saying, "I am sorry to meet you under these circumstances." It was the exact greeting I had received from the first breast surgeon. I was thinking to myself, "I am scared, and I am not pleased to meet you. This is a lot." However, with a forced smile and low enthusiasm, I said hello and introduced my niece. Displaying low energy is the opposite of who I am as a person. I subscribe to the belief that my attitude is my life. It is my nature to smile and be enthusiastic throughout the day. People tell me that my passion for life is contagious. But that day, I was struggling to be that girl.

The surgeon was nice and her confident walk and presence commanded respect and exuded power. She wore heels, and her hair was in a neat bun. Although Dr. Styles was candid and serious, she was compassionate and relatable. I was glad that a cookie-cutter approach to treatment and care wasn't her style.

She took the time to understand my personality, the specifics of my cancer, and listened to and respected my input.

Dr. Styles shared most of the same breast cancer information I had received earlier in the week from Dr. Stallone. Also, she had the second pathology report that described the biology of my cancer because an Emory pathologist had examined my tumor specimen prior to my visit. As you probably know, I didn't want to hear more "bad news." I thought, "There is no way I have triple-negative breast cancer like my Aunt Addie." Why did I think I was exempt from getting an aggressive type of breast cancer?

All breast cancer is a serious disease, but some triple-negative breast cancer (TNBC) subtypes can be very aggressive and deadly. As I explained earlier, TNBC is not supported by female hormones, or by the overexpression of HER2 receptors. Moreover, TNBC is an aggressive breast cancer subtype that disproportionately affects BRCA1 mutation carriers and young women of African origin. There is evidence that African-American women with TNBC have worse clinical outcomes than women of European descent.[1]

On that awful day, Dr. Styles uttered the words I dreaded: "Ms. Bass you have triple-negative breast cancer in your right breast."

"What did you say?" I thought. I was speechless. There was a sudden sharp pain in my chest, and I almost started hyperventilating. Instead, I looked over at my niece, who pretended to write in a notebook. She avoided eye contact and kept her head down. Laquisha was trying to be strong for her Auntie Quita, but I knew she was distraught. If we had made eye contact, both of us would have become unglued. So, we tried to remain calm by avoiding eye contact and not speaking. For a moment, I felt like I was, once again, in the *Twilight Zone*.

I broke the silence by announcing, "I am going to have a bilateral mastectomy. My Aunt Addie referred me to you, and she is a patient here. She has triple-negative breast cancer that has metastasized to her brain, so there is no way I am going to keep my breasts."

"My breasts are going to kill me" was the only thing I could think of. The breast surgeon rolled her chair in front of me and looked straight into my eyes and said in a soothing tone, "*You have to have your own experience.*"

I thought, "How in the world does she expect me to *have my own experience* when my aunt is dying from the EXACT cancer she is telling me I have?"

Dr. Styles continued, "Your tumor is very small, and you are healthy, other than the cancer. I have seen patients who have been cured of triple-negative breast cancer."

I thought, "No shit. Everyone I personally know with TNBC is dead or is dying."

If I had allowed one teardrop to leave my eyeballs, I would not have been able to stop crying, so I silently fought back tears. My emotions ricocheted from wanting to pass out on the floor to wanting to scream at the top of my lungs. Yet, I managed to maintain my composure. The triple-negative breast cancer diagnosis was the second most devastating experience of my life. My mother's death when I was a rising college senior was the first.

Emory Winship Cancer Institute is designated as a National Cancer Institute, and the location was much closer to my home than the breast care facility, so I asked Dr. Styles to perform my breast surgery. Please understand that I would have flown to Timbuktu for quality care. I have met women who crossed state lines or traveled to Atlanta from other countries to receive quality care. I was fortunate that Atlanta has a lot of renowned and quality breast cancer surgeons. I would not have gone wrong with either breast surgeon.

Decision #2 - What local treatment will I have?

Local treatment refers to how the breast tumor will be removed. When it comes to breast cancer, more aggressive breast cancer and larger tumors may require more aggressive treatment, so sometimes patients receive chemotherapy prior to surgery called neoadjuvant therapy. According to the National Institutes of Health, the purpose of administering chemotherapy before surgery is to:

- Reduce the size of the primary tumor.
- Allow an early evaluation of clinical efficacy.
- Collect relevant neoadjuvant trial results that may assist physicians to apply optimal treatment for patients with breast cancer.[2]

Furthermore, during local treatment, a patient will have either a lumpectomy, which is where the tumor is removed, or a mastectomy to remove one or both breasts. Both surgeries can be followed by radiation.

Mastectomy versus Lumpectomy

Although overall survival for lumpectomy and mastectomy are equivalent, according to the National Center for Biotechnology Information, about 5 to 10% of breast cancer patients will have local or loco-regional recurrence after breast-conserving surgery and radiotherapy within ten years of first being diagnosed with breast cancer. If the breast was removed in the course of initial treatment, cancer will reoccur in the armpit of about 5% of women or in the chest wall within ten years.[3]

During conversations about surgery options, doctors highlight that the overall survival rate for breast-conserving surgery and mastectomy are equivalent, especially for early stage breast cancer. I get it—most women want to keep their girls. Yet, it is important that patients who opt for lumpectomy and radiation understand that they are at a higher risk of having a local recurrence or a second breast cancer in the remaining breast tissue, and thus may end up having a mastectomy, after all. The risk of cancer recurring after lumpectomy is higher than after mastectomy, according to Breastcancer.org. However, local recurrence can be treated successfully with mastectomy.[4] Please listen carefully: I am not advocating for either surgery.

In 2018, my cousin Wanda experienced a recurrence seven years after she had a lumpectomy and radiation for hormone receptor-positive breast cancer which was DCIS (the cancer had not traveled outside her milk ducts). She was horrified when a tumor showed up on her mammogram because she had not understood her risk for developing a local recurrence after she finished treatment. A local recurrence is when the original breast cancer returns near the site of the original tumor.

I had the unfortunate experience of watching my cousin deal with her recurrence and witnessed the agony she went through as she scheduled her bilateral mastectomy. It was emotionally devastating for me—her cancer recurrence reminded me of my initial diagnosis. I was speechless when I heard her say on the phone, "Cousin, my cancer has returned." I was at work so all I could do was return to my desk and cry as I thought over and over in my head, "How has her cancer returned?" I was numb for the remainder of the day.

Breast cancer survivors are also at higher risk for getting another breast cancer, according to the American Cancer Society.[5] The second cancer may be unrelated to the first cancer, a fact that should be taken into consideration when deciding on surgical options. The second cancer can occur in the irradiated breast or in the opposite breast. Breast cancer that occurs in the opposite breast, after an initial breast cancer diagnosis, is called contralateral breast cancer (CBC). In an MD Anderson research study, *Mammographic Breast Density Is Associated With the Development of Contralateral Breast Cancer,* the authors concluded: "In women with primary BC (breast cancer), mammographic BD (breast density) appears to be a risk factor for the development of CBC."[6] The authors also stated that "young age at the time of diagnosis of primary BC, family history of BC, estrogen receptor–positive primary tumor, and BRCA mutation are known risk factors for developing CBC."[7]

I read a blog post written by Patricia Prijatel about the risks of getting a second cancer after a lumpectomy. She is the author of the book *Surviving Triple-Negative Breast Cancer,* and was initially diagnosed in 2006. She opted to have a lumpectomy with radiation, and chemotherapy. Unfortunately, a second primary tumor, albeit small, showed up on her mammogram in 2015.

In her blog post, she wrote, "It was in the same breast as the last one, so I could not have a lumpectomy, as that breast has already been radiated; radiation only works once. Still, I would have chosen a double mastectomy even if a lumpectomy had been an option. I would have done this with my first diagnosis had I been better informed. (Lumpectomies plus radiation are as effective as mastectomies on treating individual tumors, but they leave breast tissue that can get a second cancer later.)"

Again, I am not advocating for one surgical procedure over another. The right decision is the surgery that a patient decides to have. However, it is always a good idea to be well informed of the advantages and disadvantages of lumpectomy versus mastectomy.

ALTHOUGH I TOLD DR. STYLES I was going to have a bilateral mastectomy, she recommended a lumpectomy followed by radiation and a breast reduction in the other breast for symmetry. Dr. Styles also wanted me to get tested for the BRCA1 genetic mutation which is linked to triple-negative breast cancer and the BRCA2 genetic mutation which is linked to other cancers. According to the American Cancer Society, on average, a woman with a BRCA1 or BRCA2 gene mutation has about a 7 in 10 chance of getting breast cancer by age 80. This risk also increases if more family members have had breast cancer.[8] If I had BRCA gene mutations, I would have had a higher probability of getting breast cancer in my left breast and/or in the breast where the initial tumor was. Also, my son would be at risk of getting breast cancer. Yes, males get breast cancer, also.

Later that evening, Laquisha and I discussed my surgery options.

"Auntie, I like the surgeon's suggestion that you have a lumpectomy and reduce the size of the left breast," Laquisha said. "You have huge breasts. The doctor can inject the fat from the breast reduction into your butt. Auntie, you know you have a flat butt. When you wake up from surgery, you could look like Jennifer Lopez!"

We looked at each other and burst into uncontrollable laughter. We laughed and talked about how pretty and talented J.Lo is. And we practiced dancing like J.Lo to take our minds off breast cancer temporarily. I laughed and danced until my stomach started hurting. My goodness, did we need something to laugh about! I think it was the first time I had laughed since I had heard the dreaded words: "It's a cancer."

It turned out that I didn't have the BRCA gene mutations; the genetic test was negative. However, I decided to pass on becoming J.Lo's twin. Instead, I stuck with my initial decision to have a bilateral mastectomy with reconstruction. I was convinced that my breasts were trying to kill me. Also, I was not mentally equipped to tackle going for quarterly mammograms and ultrasounds to screen for breast cancer. The anxiety would have been unmanageable.

As recently stated, it is imperative that a patient makes her own choice about whether or not to have a lumpectomy versus a mastectomy. What a woman *decides to do* or *not do* with her body is her own business and nobody should judge her. I was thankful that Dr. Styles respected my decision to have a mastectomy, and she continued to be supportive and caring.

After I decided what surgery I would have, I was astonished to discover that other people had strong feelings about my cancer diagnosis. Some people shared their unsolicited opinions and comments with me, even after I had the surgery. A high school classmate said, "You have talked about getting a breast reduction for years, now you don't have to worry about it." Her comment was shocking and hurtful, so I remained silent. Obviously, her sensitivity chip was malfunctioning.

When I shared my breast cancer diagnosis and my treatment decision with my son, he didn't have any concept of what cancer was. His first question was, "Why can't you just take a pill to cure the cancer, and keep your breasts?" I explained to him that cancer cells are deadly and typically the first step is to remove the malignant tumor with surgery. Christopher paused, looked at me and said, "Okay Mom." Next, he walked over to his drum set and started hitting his cymbals, snare, and bass drums, playing different genres of music from his favorite musicians. Playing drums helped my son cope with the bad news. So, I sat in the living room and watched him play while I silently pleaded with God to allow me to see him pursue his musical dreams.

Jerome, my ex-husband, said, "Your breasts are your *best quality*. Why are you going to cut them off?" Furthermore, he suggested that I have a lumpectomy or ask the doctor if she could use a laser to zap the tumor. He said, "I have done research, and keeping your breasts is a viable option." I was flabbergasted by Jerome's *best quality* comment when I was fighting for my life. How dare he?

I politely responded with an eye roll, "I am comfortable with my decision. But thank you for your concern."

Breast cancer patients have to make tough decisions about surgical options. Often, the decision is extremely painful. Some women define themselves by their looks and their breasts may play a major role in how they perceive themselves and their sexuality. *I was that girl!!!* It took me a long time to admit that

I was vain when it came to my breasts. I had naturally large and voluptuous breasts, and I loved them. I liked the sexual tricks I could play with my girls. I liked to look at and touch my breasts. Each day when I stepped out of the bathtub, I used to look at myself in the large mirror facing my tub and admire my breasts. To this day, I have not gotten into my bathtub since I had my surgery in 2012: showers only. This is a painful revelation.

Decision #3 – Who will be my plastic surgeon?

Dr. Styles routinely worked with the same plastic surgeon during surgery, Dr. Lasken. Therefore, the decision was made for me. Whereas if I had gone with the first breast surgeon, I would have had to choose a plastic surgeon from the recommendations she gave me. I was relieved that selecting a plastic surgeon was one less tough decision to make.

A word of caution: should you have to pick a plastic surgeon, please get references from breast surgeons, other medical professionals, and breast cancer patients. Patients are the most important group because they can show you the finished product. Furthermore, take the time to interview multiple surgeons. During the interview ask about her experience and specialties, follow-up procedures in the event of post-surgical emergencies, and focus on her communication skills. You do not want to augment the pain from dealing with breast cancer with a bad breast reconstruction experience, if you can avoid it. Most women have positive outcomes after reconstruction surgery; however, I have met women who have had problems and complications. Some problems I have heard of include pain around the implants, swelling, and muscle spasms around the implants.

Breast reconstruction can take the form of getting saline or silicone implants, or transferring fat from other parts of the body to reconstruct new breasts. All of the procedures are complicated; each one may require a different set of skills and training. Consequently, it is imperative that your plastic surgeon is well trained for the procedure you elect to have.

According to breastcancer.org, once you have the names of a few plastic surgeons, check to make sure they meet the following criteria:

- They are certified by the American Society of Plastic Surgeons, which offers a searchable directory online. Certification means they have completed specialized training and education in plastic surgery. You can further verify their certification through the American Board of Medical Specialties. There are many surgeons out there practicing plastic surgery who are not certified, so you'll want to check on this.
- They accept your health insurance and are willing to work with your insurance provider as needed if any questions arise.
- They are available to meet your preferred time frame.[9]

Because I was eager to have my surgery as soon as possible, Dr. Styles took the extraordinary step and called the plastic surgeon while he was on vacation to ask him to come in and meet with me. Thankfully, Dr. Lasken agreed; so, my niece and I met with him the following week. As we waited for him, Laquisha and I engaged in small talk and made more jokes about me looking like J.Lo after surgery (in my dreams). Laquisha suggested that I ask Dr. Lasken if he could take some of her body fat if I needed it. As my niece and I were laughing, there was a faint knock on the door and a tall and handsome doctor walked into the room and introduced himself. He explained that he was originally from South Africa and he routinely worked with my breast surgeon and another nationally renowned breast surgeon in Atlanta.

I told him, "I am worried about getting tissue expanders before my permanent breast implants." Tissue expanders are used to stretch the skin before the permanent implants are inserted. Dr. Lasken replied, "You are a good candidate for direct implants: you are healthy, a non-smoker, have large breasts that will be smaller, and might not require radiation." He felt confident that he would be able to preserve enough breast skin to cover the implants, so I could skip the tissue expanders.

Dr. Lasken answered my questions without hesitation, had a lot of experience, was compassionate, and had a sense of humor. When my niece asked him if she could donate some of her body fat so he could build me some new breasts, he responded, "Are you twins?"

We all laughed and later met again on the elevator. I was his only patient that day because he was on vacation. It speaks volumes when a plastic surgeon comes into the office while on vacation to meet with a patient.

It is also a good idea to research physical therapists who have experience working with breast cancer patients. Your plastic surgeon will have to write a prescription in order for your insurance to cover physical therapy.

I received physical therapy at TurningPoint Breast Cancer Rehabilitation from a wonderful woman, Jill Binkley, PT, MSc, CLT, FAAOMPT, who founded the organization. During our physical therapy sessions, she engaged in conversations with me that showed that she was also concerned about my emotional wellbeing. I remember thinking, "Wow, Jill understands my emotional devastation." According to myturningpoint.org, "As a breast cancer survivor, Jill is a passionate advocate for increased attention to the unmet physical and emotional side effects of breast cancer treatment and the role of rehabilitation and exercise in improving the quality of life of breast cancer survivors." Without physical therapy, I am not sure if I would have regained my ability to lift my arms above my head and my complete range of motion after my surgery.

Decision #4 – How much time will I take off work?

My company had a generous medical leave policy; therefore, I was able to take off 13 weeks with full pay. Initially, I was scheduled to take six weeks off for recovery which is the typical recovery time for a mastectomy. The added weeks were necessary due to a second surgery three weeks after my first surgery for a breast hematoma, a blood-filled swelling that is actually a large "bruise" in the breast.

Other factors may play a role in the length of time a patient takes off work: including complications from surgery, financial stress and hardships, and fear of telling senior male colleagues about their breast cancer. I have met breast cancer patients who are senior executives in their organizations, who elected to return to work two weeks after a bilateral mastectomy with reconstruction. That is amazing.

The amount of time a person takes off work is a personal decision. For me, it was important to take enough time to recover physically and mentally. Treatment for any type of cancer can disrupt a person's family and work life. Many women may experience stress and even depression after surgery, which may require additional leave to address mental health concerns.

Decision #5 – Who would take care of me and Christopher post-surgery?

I was single when I was diagnosed, but I had a network of friends and neighbors who were very supportive. My friends Louis and Pat transported Christopher to summer camp. Also, Jerome and I were co-parents; therefore, I didn't have to worry about our son's care. Please put a support system in place prior to surgery whether you are married or single. You will need a village to help you get through the experience. If you feel like you don't have anyone, please talk to a social worker at your hospital about organizations that assist breast cancer patients. This is not the time to be a super-person and risk injury.

Most importantly, if you know a person who has had any type of cancer surgery, *please, please, please* don't tell them to call you if they need something. The statement is a cliché and useless. A lot of patients will not ask for help. Even if the person has a husband, a partner, or a large support system, she/he may still need help. The husband or partner may need to take a break; it takes a village. The cancer patient will need help with a thousand things: meals, housekeeping, laundry, transporting their kids, transportation to the doctor, yard work, running errands, babysitting, caring for pets, caring for aging parents, picking up medication, or just someone to talk to.

Don't tell them to call.

Just Show Up, Ready to Serve!

*"Lord, I am going to hold steady on to You, and
You've got to see me through."*
~ HARRIET TUBMAN

Preparing for Surgery: Battlefield in My Mind

BY THE TIME I had finished making so many tough and life-changing decisions about how I was going to proceed with treatment, I felt like I was on an emotional rollercoaster. Now, it was time to prepare for my bilateral mastectomy with reconstruction. I had good days, and I had bad days. Sadly, most days I felt the same as I had during the emotional storm that had engulfed me following my initial diagnosis: I was trying to wade my way through a freaking tsunami named triple-negative breast cancer (TNBC).

It's a cancer that is aggressive and frequently has a poor prognosis. As I mentioned earlier, I had already observed its devastation, and in my experience, most women had not survived metastatic triple-negative breast cancer.

According to an article published in *Clinical Breast Cancer,* patients in whom metastatic disease develops have a very poor prognosis, with a median survival of approximately one year.[1]

When I went to bed at night, I had conversations in my head about TNBC that I could barely control or shut down. Then I would start breaking out in hives. The itchy hives put me in a state of panic. To calm down, I prayed and asked God to stop the conversations in my head so I could fall asleep. I needed to rest because I was tired. In the infamous words of the late Fannie Lou Hamer, I was "sick and tired of being sick and tired." My options to help me sleep were prayer or drink wine, so I opted for the former. I should have chosen both options; pray, then drink wine—the entire bottle. Why didn't I ask the doctor for a sleep aid? When I opened my eyes each morning, triple-negative breast cancer was the first thought that popped into my head.

My internal mental battle was intensified as I had family and friends who were dealing with or who had died from breast cancer. This insidious disease appeared in my life like an unwelcome guest who kept showing up for dinner. As I was diagnosed, my Aunt Addie was battling metastatic triple-negative breast cancer. The horrible disease typically spreads to either the brain, liver, or lungs. My aunt's kiss of death: brain metastasis.

A breast cancer patient's worst nightmare, after the initial diagnosis and treatment, is learning that cancer has returned and spread to other body organs. No standard-of-care therapy exists for patients with metastatic triple-negative breast cancer, and therefore they have an **unmet need**.[2] Since my diagnosis, the FDA has approved treatments for metastatic TNBC. I discuss current treatments in Chapter 9.

THE WEEK BEFORE MY surgery, I visited Aunt Addie in the hospital. Nothing could have prepared me for how she looked when I stopped at the hospital door and stared at her. Addie was completely bald with a large square white bandage covering the reservoir put in place to administer chemo. My initial thought was what in the world is going on with my aunt? I can't handle looking at the person lying in the bed. I will *always* carry that image of her lying in the hospital bed in my head.

Immediately, I wanted to turn around and scream "NOOO" as I ran down the hall to leave the hospital as quickly as I could. Then, my son nudged me from behind to force me to enter the room. Addie could sense that I was in total shock, so she forced a huge smile and said, "It's great to see you Marquita and Mr. Christopher." She loved my son and was very proud of his musical accomplishments, so she would affectionately call him Mr. Christopher.

My lips were sealed, so I didn't respond when Addie said, "Hi." I couldn't speak. Addie's doctors had warned her about the risks and the small probability of a positive outcome after receiving chemotherapy to her brain. Addie didn't care how small a chance she had — she had unfeigned faith. This is why she had the courage to allow doctors to implant a reservoir in her head for chemo. My aunt was a fighter like Muhammad Ali, a trait I have seen in so many breast cancer patients. Our strength and fierce desire to live are incredible.

When my aunt told me she was going to get chemo drugs in her brain, I thought, "Why hasn't my aunt decided that she has had enough chemotherapy, and now it is time to focus on making the most of each day? When is *Enough Chemotherapy, Enough Poison*? Why doesn't she focus on the quality of her life and living, instead of trying not to die?" Actually, I didn't have to understand the choices my aunt was making. She was at peace with her treatment, that is what mattered. So, I never shared with her my thoughts about stopping chemo.

Christopher appeared to be oblivious to how Addie looked. He said, "Hi," and stood quietly in a corner. I sat in a chair facing her and silently asked the questions, "Is my destiny staring me in the face? Am I going to end up like my aunt?"

Then I started thinking, "This is some scary shit." The racing thoughts triggered slight heart palpitations, so I struggled to hold a conversation. Other family members were in the room talking and laughing, and I didn't hear a word. Darn! I had returned to that place again, the *Twilight Zone*. Somehow, I managed to remain seated in the chair throughout the visit without going into cardiac arrest.

My son did not say anything as we walked to the car. I was wondering if he was thinking about how things were going to turn out for his mom. My goal was not to burden or upset him with my disease, so I started a conversation about his favorite topic: music. We talked about the Julliard and Georgia State University summer music camps that he was going to attend. All was well in his world, I assumed.

TWO DAYS BEFORE SURGERY

On the morning of June 11, 2012, I woke up early feeling anxious and sad. Although I appeared and *acted* as though I was okay and in control when I was around others, I was emotionally distraught. Everyone, including my doctors, kept repeating, "Have your own experience with the disease. The statistics about breast cancer outcomes relate to a group, not to an individual. You are healthy." I thought, "How in the proverbial place below am I supposed to do that?" I needed more inspiration than words.

My schedule was slammed; I had so much to take care of before my surgery. In two days, I would be lying on an operating table while a breast surgeon removed my breasts, followed by a plastic surgeon popping in two silicone balls as replacements. Visions of the process remained in my head, and it was so freaking surreal. Why was this happening to me?

My typical morning routine included watching *Good Morning America* while I walked on the treadmill. I enjoyed watching *Good Morning America's* cast, especially Robin Roberts. Ms. Roberts had been popular on the Atlanta scene when she was on the radio station V-103. Now she is an anchor on a popular national morning show with a major network. This talented woman has risen from radio to ESPN to *Good Morning America*. I am super proud of her.

Instead of watching television, I decided to just walk so I

could focus on my cancer diagnosis, surgery, and the road ahead of me. While I was on the treadmill, I asked God the same questions over and over, *"How am I supposed to have my own breast cancer experience and not allow the breast cancer stories that are around me to color and shape my thinking? How am I supposed to do that?"*

My Aunt Addie was dying from metastatic TNBC cancer that started as early stage cancer like I had. Also, my sweet and lovely neighbor of 20 years, Valerie, had died from triple-negative breast cancer three years before my diagnosis. Boy, I was struggling to have my own experience.

Then, I had an epiphany: Robin Roberts had been treated for triple-negative breast cancer, and she has survived and endured chemotherapy. She appears to be thriving and healthy. Suddenly I became extremely excited and encouraged. At that moment, I almost turned on the television to watch *Good Morning America* to look at her. Instead, I kept walking, thinking, and praying.

I had followed Ms. Roberts during her breast cancer journey, so I knew she had undergone a lumpectomy, radiation, and chemotherapy treatments. I thought, "Wow, she looks fabulous! My experience may not turn out badly after all." Although I had followed Ms. Roberts cancer journey, I never took the time to understand the potentially deadly disease, TNBC. I write this with tears in my eyes, I didn't even make an effort to understand triple-negative breast cancer when my Aunt Addie was diagnosed. Her cancer recurrence, two years after her initial treatment, sparked my interest. Talk about destiny. There I was, fighting TNBC. It was freaking unbelievable!

Robin Robert's cancer journey gave me hope for the first time since I had heard the horrifying and heart-wrenching words, "You have triple-negative breast cancer." She appeared to be in excellent health, and her success encouraged and helped me accept the fact that I was going to have chemotherapy. Chemo is the only initial treatment for TNBC cancer before or after surgery. My goal was to survive and thrive like Ms. Roberts. I was so excited that I planned to email her after my surgery to introduce myself and tell her how she had given me hope. Unfortunately, I never wrote the email.

After I finished my workout, I rushed out of the house to run last-minute errands. During a doctor's visit, the nurse told me to avoid contact with sick people. She said, "The surgeon will not operate if you show any signs of a cold or any illness, and you definitely can't have a fever."

Also, a person's immune system is the first line of defense against disease, so I couldn't afford to have a compromised immune system. Therefore, I ate a lot of fruits and vegetables, stepped up my exercise routine, and attempted to get a lot of rest. Two out of three was not bad. I didn't get enough sleep.

Visiting the braid shop was my last errand. To my dismay, a family member had not responded to my request to braid my hair at her home. Oh well, I had to go to the braid shop. It was a Monday, so the shop was not crowded, which made me feel at ease because I wouldn't be around a lot of people.

As I was getting my hair braided, I received a phone call from a friend who started talking about her son's challenges with his grades at school. She was going on and on about her problems and how upset she was. "What do you think I should do?" she asked. My silent answer was, "*I am neither emotionally nor mentally equipped to have this conversation right now. I am going through one of the most devastating experiences of my life. Frankly, I don't care about your problems.*"

This thought was so out of character for me. Although I tried to be sympathetic and engage in the conversation, I did not have an answer to her question. All I could do was politely make up an excuse to end the phone call.

If ever there was a time when I couldn't be everything to everybody, this was the time. Family and friends blow my phone up when they want advice or need help. However, when things are going well for people, my phone hardly rings, "just to say hello." For some reason, I wasn't aware of this dynamic until I found myself often alone during the latter days of my recovery. There were few phone calls or visits: just me alone. It was a life-changing realization that I am still struggling to reconcile, seven years later.

After I finished talking to my friend, I struggled to remain calm and not lose my mind. It was difficult. The stylist who was braiding my hair was talking to a coworker who had a cold; I couldn't believe it. The coworker was coughing, sneezing, and blowing her nose. It may have been my imagination, but I thought I felt the lady breathing on me.

Panic, fear, and concern for my health consumed my mind. I wanted the lady to leave until the stylist was finished with my hair. She wasn't working on a client anyway. The breast surgeon was not going to operate if I had any signs of a cold. My breast cancer was aggressive, and I needed to have surgery in two days.

Prayer is my primary solution when I need help right away.

"God, please, please, help me stay seated in this chair and not give in to my instincts to jump up and run out of this shop as fast as I can," I prayed.

I would not be able to lift my arms above my head for a few weeks after surgery, so I needed braids. As I prayed, I could faintly hear the following devastating news in the background on the television. It was unbelievable. Diane Sawyer was on the news, and she said some variation of these words.

"Robin Roberts announced this morning she has been diagnosed with Myelodysplastic Syndrome (MDS). MDS is a rare blood and bone marrow disease. It may have been caused by chemotherapy."

Robin Roberts has MDS? "It may have been caused by chemotherapy," played over and over in my head. My heart felt like it had stopped beating, ejected itself from my chest, and landed in my lap. All of a sudden, there was silence.

I could not hear the sounds from the television.

I could not hear the sounds of the lady's cough.

I could not hear anything.

Suddenly I wanted to scream, *"Oh my God! Robin Roberts, why is this happening to you?"* I was in total disbelief and shock. Ms. Roberts had come to mind as an inspiration earlier that morning because she had survived triple-negative breast cancer and chemotherapy. Now, she has MDS. I asked myself, *"What in the hell is MDS?"* I don't know why I didn't Google it on my phone.

Instead of screaming and possibly passing out, I started praying.

> *"God, please give Robin Roberts strength to handle the diagnosis even though I don't know what it is. Why is this happening to her? God, I am sad for Ms. Roberts. How can this be happening when earlier I had the revelation that she was my inspiration to thrive through my journey?"*

My goodness, Ms. Roberts was the *only* TNBC cancer survivor I had heard of who had not had a recurrence. Her MDS diagnosis devastated me.

Surprisingly and miraculously, I was soon able to answer the questions I was asking God.

As I sat in the chair, I remembered a book recommended to me by a chaplain at the hospital where my mom died from pancreatic cancer. I had gone to the chaplain for prayer and support. I was trying to make sense of why my mom was dying from cancer at 49. She was the most God-fearing, loving, resilient, and unselfish person I knew.

The book is *When Bad Things Happen to Good People* written by Rabbi Harold S. Kushner. As I asked God, *"Why is this happening to Robin Roberts?"* I remembered how Rabbi Kushner addressed a similar situation in his life when his son Aaron died from a rare disease at a young age. "The question should not be, 'Why did this happen?' Instead, the question should be, 'Now that this has happened, what am I going to do about it?'"

After reflecting on the book, I added the following items to my "To Do" list.

- Pray for Robin Roberts every day as she goes through her journey
- Research MDS
- Research TNBC and Chemotherapy

On my way home from the braid shop, I called Aunt Addie. I shouted, "Have you heard the news about Robin Roberts?"

"Calm down, I thought about you as soon as I heard the news. I know the oncologist will recommend chemo, but you will be fine," she said in a low voice.

"But, no, Ms. Roberts is the only person I know who hasn't had a cancer recurrence after treatment, and I just decided this morning that she is my vision of hope," I said. Then, I immediately felt like a jerk and insensitive. My aunt was dying, and I was venting about my concerns. Dang! I guess my sensitivity chip was malfunctioning.

"Please calm down and pay attention to the road. You will be fine," Addie assured me.

Well, I was scared, so I rushed home to research MDS. According to the Myelodysplastic Syndromes (MDS) Foundation, MDS are a group of diverse bone marrow disorders in which the bone marrow does not produce enough healthy blood cells. MDS is often referred to as a "bone marrow failure disorder." Radiation and chemotherapy for cancer are among the known triggers for the development of MDS. Patients who take chemotherapy drugs or who receive radiation therapy for potentially curable cancers, such as breast or testicular cancers, Hodgkin's disease, and non-Hodgkin's lymphoma, are at risk of developing MDS for up to 10 years following treatment, according to the MDS Foundation.[3]

Thank you, Robin Roberts, from the bottom of my heart for sharing your tragedy with the world two days before my surgery. Your unfortunate life-threatening MDS diagnosis experience propelled me to research TNBC and chemotherapy after my surgery. I am so sorry you had to go through the horrific experience. You were in my heart and prayers daily during your MDS journey. I cried and agonized when you were sick after your bone marrow transplant. I watched how fragile and weak you looked when you were confined to your apartment. I watched your coworkers in masks when they visited you. Even now, I become concerned if you look like you are under the weather, a rare occurrence, while on camera. Being the winner that you are, you have come out on top again after dealing with another deadly disease. I thank God and rejoice that you are alive and well.

THE NIGHT BEFORE MY SURGERY

Praise God! I didn't catch a cold. The night before surgery, I spent quiet time reading poems from *Just for You* by Helen Steiner Rice, a book from my mom's collection. I missed my mom as I was going through my journey, so I felt close to her as I read the book. As I read the inspirational poems and prayed, I felt mentally, emotionally, and physically prepared for the Grand Finale, Day of Surgery. God transformed my whimsical emotions from feeling as though I were wading through a tsunami to feeling as though I had risen above the waves and survived.

Rice's words were encouraging, soothing, and faith-centered. Rice's poem, *God Knows Best,* gave me the most comfort because she talked about crying. Up to that point, I didn't cry much and *acted* like I was okay even when I felt like a massive pile of horse poop. The poem gave me permission to acknowledge my fear of not waking up from surgery, to embrace my grave concern that I might leave my son when I was just 48 (a year earlier than my mom died from pancreatic cancer), and to be mad and sad about having breast cancer, especially the type with a poor prognosis.

A waterfall of tears poured from my eyes. The experience was cathartic and necessary. I wiped my eyes, blew my nose, and exhaled, praying,

> *"God, please, release more than twelve legions of angels to protect me and surround me during surgery. I am tired and weary."*

Instantly, I felt the Spirit of the Lord, and I felt comforted. It was a spiritual encounter that I will never forget. I slept for seven straight hours that night, the most rest I'd had since my diagnosis.

CHAPTER 5

*For God has not given us a spirit of fear, but of power
and of love and of a sound mind.*
~ 2 TIMOTHY 1:7, THE BIBLE (NEW KING JAMES VERSION)

The Bipolar Patient

I AWOKE ON JUNE 13, 2012, rested and ready for surgery. Boy, I needed those seven hours of sleep. Before my alarm went off, I jumped out of bed and hopped on my treadmill. As I walked and prayed, I felt energized and eager to get through the operation. Next, I soaked in the bathtub, which would be the last time I soaked in a bathtub.

Thinking back, the deep sadness that consumed me for months after my surgery started that morning. The sadness began when I stepped out of the bathtub and realized that I would never look like "the girl" in the mirror again. I grabbed my cell phone and took pictures of my breasts as I admired them in the mirror. Please don't judge me. I liked my breasts, I was vain, and I wanted pictures. On the other hand, I have only looked at those pictures once since my surgery. For a brief moment, I considered texting the pictures to my ex-husband. The thought went away as soon as I remembered his comment, "Your breasts are your best quality; why are you going to cut them off?" I was fighting for my life, and I didn't care about my ex-husband's opinions about my body. I refused to be crushed by his fantasies about me. No pictures for him!

At 6 a.m., my niece Tomika arrived to take me to Emory University hospital for my surgery scheduled for 9 a.m. When we got there, a hospital representative told us the doctor was still in an earlier operation that had run over. During the wait, my family members who met us at the hospital did everything possible to remain upbeat and positive. While other families sat quietly and didn't interact much, my family laughed and talked a lot. No one appeared to be sad or concerned about my surgery. We cracked jokes, reminisced about past funny events, and tried to avoid the topic of cancer. Aside from being a little sad and very hungry, because I had not eaten anything since 6 p.m. the night before, I was okay.

Finally, at about 11 a.m., I was dressed in a blue hospital gown and waiting to be moved into the operating room. Dr. Styles, my breast surgeon, was the first doctor to show up to speak with me. She assured me that I would be okay and rolled her eyes at the nurse who claimed she couldn't find my chart and the extra pillow I had requested. Dr. Styles walked away and returned with my chart. She was no-nonsense, but professional. Dr. Styles is a bad-boss doctor, in the good sense. And, yeah, her hair was in a bun, and she had on heels. I loved her: she was smart, confident, and compassionate. Our interactions were very positive, so I felt upbeat and optimistic after she left.

Dr. Lasken, my plastic surgeon, showed up with a big smile on his face and color markers in his pocket. As he drew lines and circles on my chest like a preschooler, he explained that he was highlighting the breast with cancer and the breast without disease. He talked as he drew. To my surprise, he drew circles around my nipples and said, "We are not keeping the nipples." My mood plummeted as fast as a car getting ready to take off on the Autobahn in Germany. I went from being upbeat and positive to feeling depressed in a split second. I suddenly felt as though I had lost control of my emotions. The reality of the journey I was on became real for me at that moment. After speaking with other breast cancer patients, I learned that these emotional fluctuations are typical. There is so much information to process, so many lab tests and scans, and so many difficult decisions to make in a short period of time. Fortunately, most patients survive the overwhelming emotional unrest and ultimately thrive down the road. I am happy that the breast cancer journey is *The Road Less Traveled* for most women.

Immediately after Dr. Lasken finished drawing on my chest, I looked down. When I saw the markings, I had to struggle to avoid a complete meltdown. I wanted to yank the IV out of my arm, jump off the bed, and run out of the hospital in my gown screaming, "Noooooo." I thought, "Heck no – this can't be real." For some reason, it never occurred to me that I would lose my nipples during the operation, and I didn't remember talking to Dr. Lasken about my nipples. When he covered what would happen with my nipples during my office visit—and he most likely did—I guess I didn't hear it. Obviously, I wasn't mentally present during that conversation. Often during doctor visits, I was in the *Twilight Zone* because my mind would wander off to a place that seemed unreal. Also, I didn't read the great notes my niece took during visits. Most days, I felt exhausted after doctor visits.

It wasn't until my plastic surgeon started drawing on my chest that the reality that I was losing my breasts, nipples, and getting breast implants truly sank into my brain. How crazy was that? The plastic surgeon turned my chest into a coloring book, and suddenly, I could see a colorful picture of what body parts I was going to lose. I freaked out in my head.

"Do you have any questions?" Dr. Lasken asked.

"Can I keep my nipples, please?" I pleaded.

"No," he replied.

My heart almost stopped beating as I thought, "Are you freaking kidding me, and why am I just now understanding this?"

As Dr. Lasken explained the reasons that my nipples had to go, the only words I heard were "large breasts" and "aggressive cancer." At that moment, I couldn't comprehend why I wasn't a candidate for nipple-sparing surgery. Dang! My mind wandered off to *The Twilight Zone* again. Surprisingly, all the exciting moves during sex I had ever made with my girls raced through my mind. *No kidding,* it was a bizarre experience, and no one around me realized what thoughts were floating around in my head. Instead of being concerned about the outcome of my surgery or whether or not I would see my son again—at that particular moment—I thought about how the operation would affect my sex life. I felt sad and devastated.

My obsession with my nipples was linked to my realization that my sex life would never be the same. After my diagnosis, I was consumed with doctor visits, making tough decisions, and making sure my child was okay. At the same time, I wanted to have as much sex as possible. I suggest getting between the sheets with your husband, partner, boyfriend, girlfriend, or friend with benefits as much as possible before surgery as a way to relieve daily stress. Also, your sex life will change, and many people won't talk about that. The change doesn't have to be bad; it's just different.

Furthermore, it may be a while before your libido returns after surgery due to pain, sadness, and depression. Depression directly affects your interest in sex.[1] Furthermore, depression is a common result of both the diagnosis and the treatment of breast cancer. Chemotherapy and hormone therapy drugs pre-scribed for treatment after surgery can also affect your sex life.[2]

More importantly, if you ever need a mastectomy, please, please, have a conversation about keeping your nipples, if you care about nipples. The nipple-sparing mastectomy technique preserves both the skin envelope and the nipple areolar complex through a barely visible skin incision in the fold where the breast meets the chest, followed by immediate breast reconstruction.[3] It is a crucial concept I wish I had paid attention to and under-stood before the day of surgery, even if I wasn't a candidate for the procedure.

The last doctor to show up for the Grand Finale, Day of Surgery, was the radiologist Dr. Stoic. He was a kind and observant doctor who appeared to have a lot of experience based on his mature appearance, poise, and intuition. Although he had missed my interaction with the plastic surgeon, he immediately recognized that I was an emotional mess and not a happy patient. I am sure he didn't realize that I was upset over losing my nipples.

The first words out of his mouth were, "How are you feeling? You appear to be stoic." I was silent and stared at him as if I hadn't heard his question, which was very rude and unlike me. In an attempt to establish a rapport with me, Dr. Stoic told me a detailed story about a family member who had survived breast cancer.

"Did she survive triple-negative breast cancer?" I thought.

I was fighting back the tears and feared I would become unhinged if I uttered one word, so I remained silent. Dr. Stoic assured me that he was going to monitor me closely during surgery and make sure I was comfortable. My mind was fixated on losing my nipples, so I found no comfort in his words, as caring and compassionate as they were.

After the radiologist reviewed my chart, he told me his assistant would be back to give me some medicine. I thought I was going to get a mild sedative so I could relax while I was waiting. A young lady who looked like she was a teenager returned and asked if she could give me the medication the radiologist ordered. You know I wanted to ask her if she was of legal age. Instead, I replied, "Yes." I don't know what type of sleep sedation drug she gave me in my IV, but it knocked me out immediately. I was thankful for the medication because I never saw the inside of the operating room.

Is it a standard practice to heavily sedate a patient before surgery? Or did the radiologist recognize that I was on the verge of a meltdown? Whatever the case, I was thankful because I might have gone into cardiac arrest if I had seen the inside of an operating room.

THE NEXT WORDS I heard were, "Ms. Bass, you are in recovery. What is your pain level?"

Holy Cow! My pain level was almost as bad as the pain I experienced giving birth to my son, which is why he is an only child. I opened my eyes, and Bruno Mars was standing over me. My handsome nurse with dark hair looked just like the famous singer and songwriter, Bruno Mars.

"I am in excruciating pain," I replied. He asked me to rate my level of pain on a scale of one to 10.

"Ten."

Although I was in excruciating pain, I felt special because it seemed like I was his only patient. He was kind, caring, and attentive, and it seemed like he never left my side. It was definitely a 24-carat experience.

Tomika was standing at my side, and she told me I had been in recovery for a while. But, the hospital didn't have a room available for me to move into yet. The handsome nurse gave me morphine, and I drifted off to sleep. After sleeping for what seemed like an hour, I woke up and saw my son, Christopher, and my ex-husband, Jerome, standing over me. My son looked worried and sad, so I pretended like I was okay. I forced myself to smile in what probably looked more like a grimace. My heart was heavy, and I wanted to cry. I was happy that I lived to see my child again. The nipples didn't matter after all. Again, I *acted* like I was okay, even though I was in excruciating pain.

I was waiting to be moved to a room and in pain, and it was a school night, so I asked Jerome to take Christopher home. I wanted my son to have time to do his homework and practice his music. Furthermore, I didn't have the energy to pretend like I was okay—the pain in my chest felt like someone was hitting me with steel boxing gloves. My ex-husband and my son left. As I said bye, I noticed sadness on their faces.

All women who have a bilateral mastectomy don't experience the same level of pain I did. Unfortunately, I have a low pain tolerance so I may have been the exception. Also, the emotional distress I had experienced prior to surgery may have contributed to my post-surgical physical pain. If you ever have this surgery, please try to get adequate rest, remain calm, and ask your surgeon to prescribe sedatives that you can take before arriving at the hospital. Don't forget to understand everything you need to know about saving your nipples (if that matters to you) before the day of surgery. It may make a difference in your mood.

After Jerome and Christopher left, I had a sudden urge to pee, so I told my nurse. He responded, "I will have to get a bedpan, you have been under anesthesia for a long time." Pride can be a bad thing. The look I gave my nurse conveyed, "There is no way I am going to use a bedpan, especially with the assistance of someone who favors Bruno Mars, so I will try to hold it."

A few minutes later, two beautiful guardian angels showed up and rolled my bed to a restroom. Can you imagine how happy I was to see those beautiful ladies? I know my nurse called them: he was a class act. One nice lady helped me to the toilet and even obliged my request to wipe it off with disinfectant so I could sit down. There was no way I was going to be able to squat after a bilateral mastectomy and level 10 pain.

Fortunately, I received outstanding post-surgical care. The recovery-room staff must pay close attention to a patient's vital signs, pain level, and progress so they can immediately address any problems. In addition to choosing the right surgeon and plastic surgeon, a patient should also research the hospital where the surgeon practices. Kind nurses and a hospital with strong operating practices play a vital role in a patient's recovery. After the operation is over, the hospital staff takes care of you. If the recovery room staff fails to recognize and report abnormal behavior or physical signs, a patient's recovery could be at risk.

Around 10 p.m., I finally was taken to a room. My niece sprayed my room down with Lysol and made sure I had bottled water. The nurse on the floor was excellent and caring. Her energy and enthusiasm were refreshing, especially because I was in excruciating pain. Also, she checked on my niece and me regularly. Can you imagine having a grumpy and unresponsive nurse after having major surgery? That would be a bad experience.

The nurse added Toradol to manage my pain, and I finally got relief. I thought I was going to die until I started receiving the Toradol; the morphine alone wasn't cutting it. Toradol is a nonsteroidal anti-inflammatory drug (NSAID) commonly used for pain before or after surgery. The pain was so intense that the slightest movement of my upper body hurt.

My Aunt Sandra and my sister, Patty, showed up and woke me up around midnight to make sure I was being taken care of and not in too much pain. Sandra is a nurse, so she poked on me, looked at my breasts, and asked if I was nauseated from the anesthesia. I replied, "Auntie, I am okay, and the pain medicine finally worked." I was grateful that my aunt and sister showed up, but all I wanted to do was sleep. I was relieved when they left after 30 minutes.

AT ABOUT 7 A.M. THE next day, Dr. Styles visited. Her first words were, "I think Dr. Lasken went too small on the implants. You didn't have small breasts before, and now they are significantly smaller. But he let me know he had discussed cup size with his patient, so I backed down."

Dr. Styles looked at Tomika and said, "Your aunt is going to be smaller than you after the swelling goes down."

Tomika and I looked at each other and laughed. I was amused and thrilled that the breast surgeon cared enough to be concerned about the cup size of my implants. Typically, the breast surgeon is solely focused on removing the tumor and doing the sentinel lymph node test. It's the plastic surgeon who focuses on reconstruction. As I mentioned earlier, Dr. Styles was very attentive and concerned about my overall health. I appreciated her.

Next, Dr. Styles said, "The tumor was 1.5 centimeters, and there is no sign of cancer in your sentinel lymph nodes." Although Tomika had shared the news with me, I was overcome with joy when I heard the information straight from the doctor.

A sentinel lymph node is the first lymph node to which cancer cells are most likely to spread from a primary tumor. Sometimes there's more than one sentinel lymph node. During a sentinel lymph node biopsy, the sentinel lymph node is identified, removed, and examined to determine whether cancer cells are present.[4] That's why I was elated at Dr. Styles' news; the best information I had received in a long time! If there was no sign that cancer had spread and the tumor was small, I hoped that the oncologist would not recommend chemotherapy.

I had gone to the restroom alone, my pain was manageable, I could walk by myself, and I felt well, so Dr. Styles released me to go home. She insisted that I get out with family and friends and not sit around the house being sad. I had not fooled her by *acting* like I was always okay. Before Dr. Styles left, I asked her about chemotherapy. She replied, "You have to meet with the oncologist for guidance on chemo." I knew the answer, but I was anxious. I couldn't stop thinking about Robin Roberts' MDS diagnosis.

Although I was glad to be going home, I was about to face bigger and more distressing challenges. I had to have the chemo talk with the oncologist.

CHAPTER 6

"The word 'happy' would lose its meaning if it were not balanced by sadness."

– CARL JUNG

My Joy Didn't Come in the Morning!

ONE OF MY MOST powerful memories is of resting my head in my grandmother's lap as she rubbed my head and spoke in a low, soothing voice. "Granddaughter, I know you are sad about losing your mom. Joy comes in the morning. I know you miss your mom, and it's hard. Just pray, granddaughter, and God will keep you."

I was 20 years old, sad over my mother's death, and struggling to complete my senior year in college.

My grandmother's words, "Joy comes in the morning," were in the back of my head after I was released from the hospital as I spent hours at night researching triple-negative breast cancer (TNBC) and chemotherapy. I had to somehow summon the strength to prepare for the chemo talk with my oncologist. There was no rest for the weary. However, I was determined to learn everything my brain could process about chemotherapy, TNBC, and MDS. There I was *again* on the internet. The World Wide Web is full of information on breast cancer from sources from across the globe. Therefore, I focused on information from credible sources like peer-reviewed journals, including *The New England Journal of Medicine, Science Daily,* and *The Oncologist.*

Night after night, I researched these questions:
- What is triple-negative breast cancer?
- What is the survival rate?
- What causes triple-negative breast cancer?
- Is chemotherapy effective for triple-negative breast cancer?
- What are the side effects of chemotherapy?
- Does chemotherapy cause MDS?

Well, "Joy" never showed up for me in the morning as I watched the sun shine through my blinds. All I felt was anger, fear, and sadness after repeatedly reading articles with titles like these.

Triple-Negative Breast Cancer: An Unmet Medical Need, Oncologist, 2011

Different Subtypes of Triple-Negative Breast Cancer Respond to Different Therapies, Science Daily, 2011.

Triple-negative breast cancer: are we making headway at least? Therapeutic Advances in Medical Oncology, 2012

Despite having higher rates of clinical response to presurgical (neoadjuvant) chemotherapy, TNBC patients have a higher rate of distant recurrence and a poorer prognosis than women with other breast cancer subtypes, Journal of Clinical Investigation, 2011

Risk of Aggressive Breast Cancer Subtype Three Times Higher for African-American Women, Science Daily, 2009

The aforementioned articles are depressing. Thank goodness, a lot of women survive triple-negative breast cancer.

The second week after my surgery, my girlfriend Shelia visited from Texas bringing information from the Gerson Institute, a non-profit organization in San Diego, California. My beautiful friend traveled to San Diego from Austin, Texas, to get information on the Gerson diet, an alternative, non-toxic treatment for cancer and other chronic degenerative diseases. Gerson recommended organic fruits, vegetables, and whole grains, so Shelia and I shopped at the health food store and the farmer's market so we could prepare healthy meals. Typically, I ate a plant-based organic diet before I was diagnosed, which obviously didn't prevent TNBC. Nevertheless, I still believe that a woman should be aware of her specific breast cancer risk factors and make an effort to manage them. Furthermore, I think my healthy eating habits and overall general health have played a role in my seven-year survival.

Shelia and I prepared healthy meals, spent time talking about relationships, and watched television when I wasn't searching for my son's socks, riding around trying to find the right-sized reeds for his saxophone, or going with my ex-boyfriend's mom to the bank to assist her with her mortgage loan closing. Even though the guy had emotionally devastated me the year before, I love his mom. So, I continued to help her.

One evening, with a concerned look on her face, Shelia said, "I am flabbergasted. You act as if you have not had surgery. You are still being supermom and extending yourself to others like you are well." I was speechless. She is my rock, incredibly smart, and eloquent. Shelia always knows what to say to help me solve difficult problems. This time, my good friend didn't know how to help me because I *acted* like I was well. Thinking back, I believed that I had to be strong and *act* normal. Otherwise, I would have become unraveled. I was so freaking scared, literally frightened of dying.

What Shelia didn't see was how I cried myself to sleep on the few nights I didn't stay up all night on the computer until daybreak. She didn't witness me standing in the shower and barely bathing. I didn't know what I was supposed to do with the freaking drains hanging from both sides of my body. After a mastectomy, you leave the hospital with tubes that come out of the incision site to collect fluids in a rubber container that is attached at the end of the tube. The drains are removed once the drainage stops.

When I was alone in my bedroom, I cried a lot. I had survived the destructive emotional storm I was in when I was diagnosed. Surprisingly, I had risen above the maelstrom I feared as I waited for surgery. After my surgery, I feared the post-surgery treatment was going to destroy the foundation of my health and kill me.

After Shelia left, it was just Christopher and me—oh boy! He was my lifeline when he wasn't with his dad. My son helped out with house chores, made my bed, and agreed to do my laundry under one condition. With a pained look on his teenage face, he blurted, "I am NOT going to touch your panties." I laughed and said, "Okay, we have a deal."

We ate meals that friends and neighbors cooked for us. My neighbors Beverly and Annie volunteered to take me to the doctor, and they dropped off healthy meals. They called or texted me almost daily, and I appreciated them. They were my guardian angels. Thank You, God! I spent my nights conducting research and my days with Christopher, so I was thankful not to have to worry about food, until it ran out.

And then the Saturday morning from hell hit us.

A few weeks had passed, and the revolving door of friends and neighbors had slowed down. That morning, my son followed me downstairs like a shadow and asked, "When are you going to get better so you can cook?" I ignored his question because I realized that the frontal lobe of his 14-year-old brain was not fully developed. He wasn't totally responsible for being immature and insensitive. Furthermore, I was not in the mood to go there with him. I was hungry, sad, and tired. I had been up all night on the computer. It was definitely a "don't mess with Mom day."

As we got downstairs, Christopher headed toward the family room, and I went to the kitchen. When I got there, I saw drumsticks on the kitchen counter.

Now, I had repeatedly told my son, "Don't leave your drumsticks on my kitchen counter. They are dirty from your sweaty palms, and they don't belong on the counter." Seeing those drumsticks hijacked my emotions. At that exact moment, my son yelled, "Mom—I am hungry."

I shifted from anger to rage. Before I had time to think, I grabbed the drumsticks with my right hand, *the side where my tumor was removed*, and threw them like I was Satchel Paige. The sticks traveled 15 feet in the air from the kitchen, across the breakfast bar, through the breakfast sitting area, and hit the fireplace in the family room where Christopher stood.

I shouted, "How many times have I told you to please keep your dirty drumsticks off my kitchen counter? Go upstairs to your room, and I don't care if you starve." Immediately, I noticed the shock and sadness on Christopher's face as he jumped out of the way. My son fought back tears and went to his room.

Ouch! I can imagine the mental health professionals writing in my chart:

> "*That behavior was not about the drumsticks and the fact that said patient was hungry and stressed; although those factors may have contributed to the erratic behavior. The patient presented with symptoms of intermittent explosive disorder, which manifests as verbal and behavioral outbursts. Said outbursts are typically out of proportion to the situation that triggered the rage.*"

Thank goodness Christopher jumped out of the way, so his temporarily insane mom didn't hit him. That would have devastated me even more. My son was my life, so I would never intentionally hit him with any object. Although I was stressed, I wasn't trying to hit my child. In the blink of an eye, I lost my mind, *finally*, and became unraveled. As I hurled the drumsticks across the room, I felt myself releasing a lot of suppressed painful emotions. From the look on my son's face, he either sensed that I needed to release my anger and exhale, or he was just in shock. He looked like a deer startled by headlights.

For me, the experience was simultaneously cathartic and devastating. For the first time in Christopher's life, I really didn't care about my son's needs. Spending nights on the computer had taken a physical and an emotional toll. I wanted to fall on the floor and cry. A nervous breakdown seemed inevitable until God intervened, and my friend Alexsa showed up at that very moment. She brought a veggie sandwich and other groceries, and she stayed to visit with me. I can't remember if I offered to share any food with my son—WOW!

During our visit, the doorbell rang. I opened the door to a police officer on my porch with a concerned look on his face. The officer was young, stern, but respectful. He asked, "Did someone call 911 and hang-up?"

Before I said no, it occurred to me that I had a hungry son upstairs who might have called the police on me. For a brief moment, I wanted to chuckle. My son got the idea to call 911 from an incident that had been recently reported in the news. A few weeks earlier, the daughter of a famous and world-renowned minister in an Atlanta suburb called the police on her father. He had allegedly choked her and hit her with a shoe. I went from feeling comical to being shocked that a police officer was at my front door.

My heart racing, I could barely speak and almost cried as I told the officer, "Maybe my son called 911 because I sent him to his room for unacceptable behavior." You know I left out the minor detail about the drumsticks, and I definitely didn't say my child may be upset and hungry. Was that cruelty to a child?

It never crossed my mind. All I thought was: I am a law-abiding citizen who is dealing with aggressive breast cancer, and going to jail isn't an option.

Most African-American parents have "the talk" with their sons about how to behave when it comes to interacting with police officers. At that moment, I was ready to send my son, who I would die for, with that nice white officer.

He asked, "How old is your son?"

"Fourteen," I replied.

"Ma'am, I need to interview your son alone. Please ask him to come outside."

I shouted upstairs, "Christopher, there is a police officer here to see you."

He emerged at the top of the stairs with fear plastered on his face. He walked outside, and I returned to my visit with Alexsa while fighting back tears. Alexsa had a dumbfounded look, wondering what in the world was going on. I don't recall what we discussed or if we just sat in silence.

Christopher returned to the house after about a half hour, and quietly said, "I apologize for raising my voice at you." I didn't ask him what he told the officer. I didn't care. I was relieved that neither he nor I were leaving the house in handcuffs. My son stayed in his room until his dad picked him up a few hours later. You know I had to call his dad, and Christopher had to go. He didn't have to leave because of his behavior. He had to leave because of my earlier behavior toward him. Although Christopher and I now laugh about that morning, at the time, I felt like a horrible mother.

I desperately needed some alone time to allow myself to experience my deep pain and sadness. I needed some alone time to pray and cry openly. I needed some alone time to digest all of the disturbing information about TNBC.

Triple-Negative Breast Cancer:
- Disproportionately affects African-American women. About 30% of all breast cancers in African-American women are triple-negative, depending on the study and the geographical area where it is conducted. (What the heck?)
- Can be an interval cancer, which means that tumors grow fast and may show up between mammograms. (Wow!)
- Patients have a relatively poor outcome. (This fact is stated in every article I read.)
- Is likely to recur two to three years after treatment. (Lord, help us!)
- Survivors who live five years have a lower chance of the cancer recurring. (Something positive, thank you!)
- Patients are more likely to be under the age 40. (So disturbing!)
- The five-year survival rate is approximately 60 to 70%, depending on the study. (This is unfortunate compared to other breast cancer types. Also, survival rates don't include recurrence and metastatic cases.)
- Doesn't have a targeted treatment. (So sad and depressing for TNBC patients.)
- Is an unmet medical need. (When will this change?)
- Is not one disease, but, comprises four or six distinct subtypes, depending on the research. The tumors have different molecular features, and each subtype reacts differently to specific chemotherapy drugs. (Are you freaking kidding me?)

A COUPLE OF WEEKS later when Christopher returned, he and I spent the rest of that summer watching every episode of the television show *Lincoln Heights* and the *Paranormal Activity* movies on Netflix. His camps were over. Christopher suggested the shows, and I enjoyed sharing the experience with him. We also had a great time as I watched him practice drumming along to YouTube videos. He insisted that I pay attention and watch him practice

As a result of throwing my son's drumsticks across the room, I started experiencing excruciating pain and bruising near my right implant. Jerome took me to the plastic surgeon, and it turned out to be a traumatic appointment. The plastic surgeon said I needed to have another surgery as soon as possible to drain a pool of blood, or hematoma, around my implant. I was too embarrassed to tell the doctor the truth, so I said I had injured myself when I tried to lift my printer. My attempt to lift the printer had only exacerbated the injury. The truth: I know throwing the drumsticks did me in. Raising my arm above my head and throwing the drumsticks with such intensity caused blood to pool around my right implant. During the same visit, the plastic surgeon removed the steri-strips from my breasts. I was not prepared for seeing horizontal scars across my breasts. I fought back tears in the doctor's office as I waited for the nurse to clean the site.

As Jerome and I left the plastic surgeon's office, I told him I needed to have another surgery to drain a hematoma. I was scared and angry at myself for sabotaging my recovery by throwing the drumsticks. As I was getting ready to tell Jerome how upset I was by the sight of my surgical scars, he interrupted me by blurting, "I still don't know why you cut off your breasts anyway. They were your best physical quality. All you had to do was remove the tumor."

His comments hit me like a ton of large concrete bricks: the big gray ones. He made the same comments to me when I was diagnosed, but I'd let them pass before. This time around, I was mad as hell.

"Fuck you. I am glad we are not married. Your comments are cruel and insensitive. How in the hell can you say that dumb shit to me? Obviously, you are having a problem with it. Get over it. I am alive, and nothing else matters to me! Damn, now I need to have another surgery, and my aunt is dying. I don't need to hear your opinion about my body." Yep—I said every single word: *in my mind*.

Instead of verbally expressing the obscenities floating around in my head, I realized that Jerome was not intentionally trying to hurt my feelings, and I remained silent. With summoned courage after a few long minutes, without crying, and in a low and cracking voice, I replied, "Well I have already had the bilateral mastectomy, and my breasts are gone. So, your comments are hurtful and don't serve a purpose."

Then I shut up.

It's uncharacteristic of me to curse at a person, so I decided to shut up although I wanted to say everything I was thinking. It's no surprise that we didn't talk much during the drive home.

Jerome asked, "Do you need to stop by the store or run other errands?"

"No, thank you."

I couldn't wait for him to drop me off at home and leave me the hell alone.

Later, after my hematoma surgery, I called Jerome and asked him to come over and cook dinner for July 4th. He came over with groceries, cooked dinner, and we ate and watched television as a family. It was all good.

MY WONDERFUL AUNT ADDIE died from metastatic triple-negative breast cancer on July 7, five days after my hematoma surgery and less than three weeks after my bilateral mastectomy. I was so traumatized by her death that I couldn't gather the strength to attend her funeral. How was I supposed to be able to attend the funeral of a person who I loved, and she had died from the very disease I was battling? That pain was so intense that I actually felt it in my chest. When people called me and told me I had to pay my last respects, I became irate. I gave my aunt her roses when she could smell them. Whenever she called me and needed a favor, I was there at the speed of light. I had given her my time and shown her love, devotion, and compassion while she was alive and could appreciate it.

The last time I saw Aunt Addie alive was after my mastectomy surgery when my nieces and I went to visit her at her home. She was weak, but lucid. At the visit, I remember saying, "See you later, Aunt Addie." I looked into my aunt's frail face, and she responded with confidence, "I will be here." She was a modern-day Job. Like Job in the Bible, she continued to believe that God was going to heal her until she took her last breath, no matter how dire her medical health was. As I walked toward the door, I fought back tears. I knew I wouldn't see her alive again.

That night, I resumed my research. I had to learn more about TNBC. I was 48, and I did not want to die and leave my son.

UNFORTUNATELY, I DIDN'T KNOW the emotional toll my breast cancer journey had on my son until four years later when he went to intensive therapy the summer after he graduated from high school. In those four years, he had never shared his feelings and fears with me. Regrettably, I don't recall ever asking him how he was doing with my diagnosis. I never asked my son if he was scared. I never asked my son these critical questions or had critical conversations with him about my disease. Erroneously, I assumed that if I *acted* like I was okay and kept his routines as normal as possible, he would be fine.

That was a major blunder for me. Unfortunately, my son experienced a significant loss when my Aunt Addie died less than a month after my surgery from the exact breast cancer his mom had. Also, Christopher's best friend and neighbor, Jordan, had lost his mom, Valerie, to TNBC. Whew … that is a lot for a teenager to handle.

I should have asked questions, taken him to a counselor, or found a support group for kids of parents with breast cancer. Christopher and my Aunt Addie were very close. She called him Mr. Christopher and continuously praised him for his musical talents. We visited her often. Addie was my confidante, and she loved and supported my child. Her husband was also very close to my son, and our relationship with her husband ended after Addie's death. How could my son be okay and not be affected?

However, the emotional trauma didn't keep Christopher from attending the prestigious Berklee College of Music the fall after he graduated from high school. Berklee, the largest independent college of contemporary music in the world, accepts only one in four applicants, so it was quite an accomplishment for him to get in!

"Don't do things to not die but do things to enhance the quality
of your life and you may be surprised
by how long you do live."
~ BERNIE S. SIEGEL, M.D.

None of This Information Makes Sense to Me!

I sat in a stupor three days after Addie died while waiting for my oncologist, Dr. Zoe. She had also been my aunt's doctor.

"Ms. Bass, I am sorry to hear about the death of your aunt," Dr. Zoe said. After I thanked her, the oncologist jumped right into explaining my surgical pathology report. It is critical information in the treatment of any cancer. A pathologist analyzes the cancer tumor removed during surgery and prepares a report about what she finds. This report either validates or negates what doctors found in earlier biopsies when only tumor samples are analyzed.

According to my surgical pathology report, my tumor was in fact TNBC, which was no surprise because two pathologists had analyzed my tumor the week I was diagnosed. The good news was that my cancer was early stage, it was less than 2 cm. *This is one time in my life when "small" was a very good thing.*

The specifics of my cancer were:

- **Tumor Origination,** Invasive/Infiltrating Ductal Carcinoma.
- **Tumor Biology**, Triple-Negative.
- **Tumor Size**, 1.5cm, approximately three-quarters of an inch (or the size of an M&M peanut).

- **Tumor Grade,** 3 (cells were growing rapidly).
- **No Node Involvement,** Cancer cells had not migrated to the three lymph nodes removed during the sentinel lymph node biopsy.

There is another cancer status called vascular or lympho-vascular invasion. A pathologist uses a microscope to examine the primary tumor and the surrounding tissue. She determines if tumor cells are in the blood vessels or lymphatic channels that lead to your lymph nodes. A patient can have vascular invasion that hasn't progressed to her lymph nodes. My pathology report specified that I didn't have vascular or lymphatic system invasion, which was fantastic news. Boy, I needed some good news.

Tumor size and vessel invasion are the best predictors for "disease-free survival (DFS) in patients with stage I breast cancer," according to a study published in the Journal of Clinical Oncology.[1] Even if a patient's lymph nodes are clear, she needs to know the status of her vascular or lymphatic system. The results may have a bearing on what treatment her oncologist recommends.

My oncologist recommended four rounds of chemotherapy. Sadly, there are no other targeted treatment options for TNBC. Even with all the progress that has been made to address hormone-positive tumors and HER2 breast cancers, TNBC is the **ONLY** breast cancer that doesn't have a targeted treatment. In other words, there has been no research since the term TNBC showed up in medical journals in 2005 that has led to significant change in National Comprehensive Cancer Network (NCCN) guidelines regarding how early stage disease is initially treated in a clinical setting.

When Dr. Zoe told me that she had arranged for the chemotherapy nurse to come in to explain to me how the chemo infusion process works, I felt like she had arranged a trip for me without my consent.

I thought, "Hold up, wait a minute! I have questions for you, please." Instead, I struggled to say, "This is a very difficult time for me—my aunt died from metastatic TNBC, and here I am dealing with early stage TNBC." Without hesitating, Dr. Zoe agreed to answer my questions.

I quickly opened up the notebook that contained my research articles and questions from my nights on the computer and started firing off questions like a criminal detective.

What subtype of triple-negative breast cancer do I have?

I knew there are four or six subtypes of TNBC, depending on the study, and that results from chemotherapy can be mixed. A subgroup of women with triple-negative disease has tumors that are extremely sensitive to chemotherapy, and there are many women for whom chemotherapy is of uncertain benefit.[2]

The doctor told me she didn't know what subtype I had. "The pathology report doesn't include tumor subtypes," she said. "That type of tumor profiling only occurs in certain clinical trials and in research."

I was horrified. I almost squealed, "WHAAAT?" Instead, I suppressed my tears and outage so that I could finish asking questions.

What do you think about Robin Robert's recent MDS diagnosis?

Dr. Zoe was familiar with Robin Robert's misfortune, but she told me the risk of getting a secondary cancer like MDS is very low and rare.

What is the probability that my cancer will not come back if I take chemotherapy, compared to if I don't take chemo?

The doctor looked at me like I had suddenly grown horns. This question was important because I had read an article that stated that TNBC is an unmet medical need. Dr. Zoe reached for her laptop and opened the program Adjuvant Online, which assesses an individual patient's risk of recurrence based on treatment options. According to the tool, if I didn't take chemo, there was a 25% probability that my cancer would recur; with chemotherapy, the risk halved to 12%. I thought that 13% advantage to be modest compared to the added toxicity of chemotherapy and its horrific side effects. On the other hand, many patients will endure chemo for any percent gain, which is their right. Again, the best treatment is the one a patient is at peace with or agrees to have. I would *never* suggest that a patient not agree to chemotherapy. A lot of patients have favorable outcomes after taking chemo.

What do you think about my medical history of neutropenia, low levels of certain kinds of white blood cells?

She said because I appeared healthy, she thought I would tolerate chemotherapy well.

What do you think about my recent CT scan that shows some possible heart abnormality? Heart toxicity can be a side effect of chemotherapy.

Glancing at my report, she said she wasn't worried about it. Her terse response made me feel like conferring with a cardiologist.

Some patients follow doctor's orders and recommendations without any questions or hesitation. I have heard of cancer patients who don't want to understand any details about their disease; they just want to get through the treatments. Guess what? I totally get that. However, that's not my approach. My family and friends make fun of me all of the time. For instance, I stopped using tampons when I heard that they can lead to toxic shock syndrome under certain circumstances. Also, I skipped birth control pills because I didn't want to disrupt my endocrine system with synthetic hormones, because I feared getting breast cancer. I didn't have any idea that some breast tumors are not hormone-positive. I have always been very over-the-top about my health. Consequently, it was important for me to fully understand my disease, available treatment options, related side effects, the consequences of all available options, and the names of all my doctors' immediate family members and their shoe sizes.

Seriously, I needed to make an informed decision about a treatment that could potentially change my life forever and/or kill me. I needed to be at peace with my treatment. It had to make sense *to me*. The words "make sense" are relative. Please hear this: what makes sense to one person may not make sense to another person. We have to stop judging each other when we disagree with or don't understand another person's actions and how they decide to approach cancer treatment. I know breast cancer patients who have been ostracized by family members instead of supported by them because they don't agree with their treatment choices. How sad and unfortunate. Cancer patients need support, not judgment. Whether a patient decides to proceed with conventional treatment, alternative treatment, integrative treatment, or no treatment is her business.

"Dr. Zoe, I have to think about proceeding with chemotherapy," I said. She asked why I had reservations. I don't recall what my response was.

In my head, I ticked off my concerns:

1. Taking chemo for TNBC is a crapshoot. I would be rolling the dice. You can't tell me my tumor subtype or which chemo is proven to work best for my particular disease. Plus, I'm concerned about my medical history with neutropenia; chemo can cause neutropenia sepsis.
2. Robin Robert's MDS diagnosis makes me nervous about the long-term side effects of chemo.
3. My aunt had chemotherapy, and she's dead. I guess the chemotherapy didn't work for her triple-negative subtype.
4. My neighbor Valerie, who was also your patient, is dead.
5. I only know the type of breast cancer I don't have. Any breast cancer that isn't hormone-positive or HER2 is dumped into one bucket and called triple-negative breast cancer, which is unfortunate. (This needs to change, NOW!)

In fairness to Dr. Zoe, both my aunt and neighbor presented with metastatic breast cancer when they saw her for the first time. Who knows? If they had been her patients initially when their tumors were less advanced, they might still be alive.

My hesitancy to agree to chemo appeared to confound Dr. Zoe, who nevertheless was cordial. Although I needed to confer with additional oncologists before I decided whether to take chemotherapy, she warned me that I had one week to decide because the efficacy of the chemotherapy diminishes with time. Dr. Zoe urged me to meet with the oncology nurse and to discuss the infusion, and I could cancel if I needed to.

My visit with the nurse was short and sweet. As the nurse talked, I had images of dead people whirling in my head. She knew about my Aunt Addie's death, so she was very sympathetic and endearing.

I thought, "Don't count on seeing me in your chemo infusion chair until I get more information."

The nurse consoled me: "Have your own experience. This is your journey, and don't be influenced by anyone." She had been a chemotherapy nurse for more than 20 years, so her comments resonated with me.

After my meeting with the nurse, I walked as fast as I could, short of sprinting, to my car. As I passed people, I struggled to maintain my composure; I felt like I was on the verge of having a nervous breakdown. For the life of me, I couldn't wrap my brain around how I was expected to take a toxic treatment for a disease that I didn't fully understand. Furthermore, the oncologist couldn't fully tell me what specific TNBC subtype I had and the best treatment.

How could Dr. Zoe effectively treat my disease? She didn't know my TNBC subtype and whether my specific tumor was or wasn't chemo sensitive. That shit was bananas! However, she was doing her job by following National Comprehensive Cancer Network (NCCN) guidelines. Oncologists have to follow NCCN Clinical Practice Guidelines (nccn.org) when they treat cancer patients. Until a targeted treatment for early stage TNBC makes it through clinical trials and is approved by the FDA, TNBC patients are stuck with chemotherapy, for the most part. Or, they can find a clinical trial.

No wonder I almost crashed into the highway median on my way home. My son's face flashed in my head. Christopher's image was the motivation for me to take control of the wheel and avoid hitting the median. Was I out of my mind from fear, frustration, and the failure of the research community to have come up with a targeted treatment for TNBC?

Overall, it was a sad and devastating day. I had so many unanswered questions about TNBC. Suzanna, a TNBC survivor who has been cancer free for nine years and whom I met online, eloquently expressed how I was feeling. While debating treatment options, she said, "The more I read, the more I realized they (the oncologists) were throwing spaghetti against the wall to see what sticks." My sentiment exactly!

In the following week, my niece Tomika drove me to consult with two additional oncologists. I almost crashed my car after the first oncology visit; therefore, my niece drove me to the doctor for a year. Both doctors were awesome! I had actually visited one of the oncologists previously to address my neutropenia illness. The last oncologist I visited, Dr. Danbowski, ended up being my regular oncologist.

My first oncologist, Dr. Zoe, is a renowned TNBC oncologist respected in her field. I didn't switch doctors because she wasn't good at her job; I switched doctors because she didn't provide the hope and nurturing that I needed to thrive. Please note, I didn't say survive; I needed to thrive as a patient. She communicated with me as if she needed me to just be the "obedient" patient and go with the flow because she knew what was best for me. I felt like Dr. Zoe was a Medical Deity, a term from Dr. Bernie S. Siegel's book, *Love, Medicine, & Miracles.*

It was vital for me to have a synergistic relationship with the person who was going to prescribe a treatment that could potentially kill me. Yes, you can die from chemotherapy, especially if you already suffer from neutropenia, which I did. Chemotherapy can attack bone marrow, suppressing the production of white blood cells.[3]

Make no mistake, I am not launching a scathing attack against oncologists and chemotherapy. *Oncologists save lives!*

Dr. Danbowski was more mature and appeared to be interested in me as a whole person. Before he uttered one word about treatment options, he took the time to learn about me as a person. He asked what I did for a living, if I was happy, and about my family. He asked questions that made me feel like he cared about my life, happiness, and how I addressed decision making. I felt valued, respected, and important. Then he drew pictures of a stick person, Patty. His pictures included graphs that explained my cancer, treatment options, and outcomes. I was amazed.

He also looked at Adjuvant Online when I asked him, "What is the chance of my cancer recurring without taking chemo?" He gave me a 35% chance of recurrence without chemo, considering my mother had died from pancreatic cancer, and my family had a history of breast cancer. Your family medical history will help medical professionals make more informed decisions about your care.

Dr. Danbowski also recommended four cycles of chemotherapy, with a variation in suggested cocktails, a.k.a. the combination of chemo drugs. Furthermore, he was very adamant about his recommendation. He used words like "zapping and destroying" cancer cells as he described how the drugs would work. I felt like my treatment was chemical warfare. Ironically, chemotherapy drugs were discovered during World War II after naval personnel were exposed to mustard gas.

Thankfully, Dr. Danbowski respected my need and desire to be a part of the decision-making process. He understood my need to fully understand my disease, and he listened to my concerns about my existing health maladies. He respected my need to live and not to just exist.

Without me asking, Dr. Danbowski explained the side effects of chemotherapy in detail:

- *Short term* - hair loss, neutropenia, nausea, vomiting, fatigue, neuropathy, hospitalization, and dark fingernails.
- *Intermediate challenges* - having the port removed and memory loss.
- *Long term* - heart toxicity and secondary cancers.

Dr. Danbowski noticed that I was agonizing. I was on the fence and not embracing chemotherapy, so I was leaning toward forgoing treatment. Therefore, to my amazement, he introduced the concept of a regret matrix. The oncologist drew a matrix similar to the following diagram.

Diagram 1

Regret Matrix			
		Treatment	
		Chemo	No Chemo
Outcome	No Recurrence	Happy Patient	Happy Patient
	Recurrence	Sad Patient	Will I be at **peace** with my decision?

For the next 24 hours, I couldn't sleep as I wrestled with deciding whether or not to undergo chemotherapy. I reviewed the side effects, uncertain benefits, and the potential benefits. Iyanla Vanzant wrote in her book, *Faith in the Valley*, "You do what you think is right, only to find out it was the worst thing you could have done." For the life of me, I didn't want to fall into that category, so I prayed, cried, and continued to research. Time was of the essence. I only had a day or so before I needed to get a port, which is how the chemo medicine gets into your system.

Then I came across an interesting 2011 article in the Journal of Clinical Investigation, *Identification of human triple-negative breast cancer subtypes and preclinical models for selection of targeted therapies.* According to the authors, doctors at the Vanderbilt University School of Medicine, "Clearly, there is a major need to better understand the molecular basis of TNBC and to develop effective treatments for this aggressive type of breast cancer. More extensive genomic, molecular, and biological analyses of TNBCs are required to understand the complexity of the disease and to identify molecular drivers that can be therapeutically targeted."[4] I read that article over and over again, and I reviewed my notes from all three oncology visits. By the way, none of the oncologists I visited mentioned that TNBC is not one disease, unless I did. This comment is not meant to be derogatory or disparaging. Why would oncologists tell patients that TNBC is NOT one disease? NCCN guidelines instruct them to treat it as a single disease? I totally get it.

In another interesting article published in 2011 in *The Oncologist,* Lisa Carey, M.D., an international breast cancer expert and Physician-in-Chief of the N.C. Cancer Hospital wrote that "Chemotherapy has certainly improved over the years, but with chemotherapy alone, the residual risk remains substantially higher, between 30% and 40%. Improving outcomes in triple-negative disease will require a better understanding of the biology and drug targets in this subtype."[5] The concept of residual disease is very significant. For instance, a patient will have a decreased chance of long-term disease-free survival after neoadjuvant chemotherapy (chemo before surgery), if she has residual disease or doesn't experience a complete pathology response.

Based on my research, chemotherapy for TNBC appeared to be experimental because oncologists were treating it as one disease, and I didn't want to be the spaghetti noodle that didn't stick to the wall. It seemed like although TNBC is not one disease, chemo is administered to all patients to see what happens before another treatment or a clinical trial is recommended. More disturbing, "Physicians cannot currently predict which patients will relapse, even after intensive chemotherapy, and which patients will have long-term disease-free survival and might do equally well with de-escalation of their chemotherapy regimen," according to the authors of *A multigene assay determines risk of recurrence in patients with triple-negative breast cancer.*[6]

One oncologist argued that I had allowed my aunt's death to impair my ability to make sound decisions. True, my aunt's death colored my thinking. More importantly, I didn't want to expose myself to the toxic side effects of chemo when the benefits were uncertain. Also, I was concerned about my history of neutropenia and heart toxicity associated with Adriamycin, or Doxorubicin, an anthracycline type of chemotherapy that is used alone or with other medications to treat several different types of cancer. Doxorubicin works by slowing or stopping the growth of cancer cells. This drug is highly toxic and red in color; patients call it "Red Devil." And what about secondary cancers like MDS?

There I was *again* staying awake all night on my computer. The experience was painful, but necessary. I prayed a lot. I asked God to order my steps, give me clarity, direction, and *PEACE*.

Thank You, God! I finally experienced "Joy" in the morning. The next morning, my extensive research and intuition led me to pass on what was behind door number one and skip chemotherapy.

More significant, my cancer was early stage, there was no vascular invasion, I had a history of neutropenia, and I believed chemotherapy would have killed me. Also, there was no way to know if the treatment would lead to disease-free survival. If I was going to die, it was not going to be from the toxicity of chemo or from recurrent TNBC that may include chemo-resistant cells. After initial treatment, chemo-resistant stem cells seemed to be a common phenomenon for some triple-negative breast cancer patients. Maybe that is why every article you read refers to TNBC as cancer with a poor diagnosis that needs a targeted treatment. Amazingly, I was at **peace** with whatever outcome was ahead of me after I made the paradigm shift from being afraid to die to focusing on living. Instead of going with the gold standard treatment for TNBC, I focused on being healthy.

It was the most difficult and painstaking decision I have ever made in my life. In my opinion, chemo for early stage

TNBC was experimental because oncologists didn't know the subtype of my tumor. Please hear what I am saying: I am only sharing my journey. I would *never* tell anyone NOT to take chemotherapy. Again, I would *never* tell anyone NOT to take chemotherapy. It saves lives! However, women have the right to make their own decision about their care.

National Comprehensive Cancer Network (NCCN) guidelines from 2012 and 2019 direct oncologists to treat TNBC with chemotherapy for all hormone receptor-negative tumors greater than 1 cm.

The authors of the study, *The Triple Negative Paradox: Primary Tumor Chemosensitivity of Breast Cancer Subtypes,* wrote that chemotherapy primarily affects relapses within the first few years after diagnosis which is when the fast-growing ER negative subtypes are more likely to relapse."[7] My interpretation of what I read: Although triple-negative breast cancer may respond initially to chemo, there is a good chance that it may recur in the first years after treatment.

So, if I only had two, three, or five years to live, I was going to continue to live my best life ever until then. I was 48, and I didn't want to leave my son, Christopher. Nevertheless, it was important for me to live in a way that made sense *to me*. Furthermore, I had always focused on serving God and others, so my living had not been in vain. More importantly, I was no longer afraid to die.

My TNBC treatment included a bilateral mastectomy with breast reconstruction, and I decided, *I was done*. Next, I had to learn how to live as a cancer survivor.

CHAPTER 8

"Tough Times Never Last, But Tough People Do!"
~DR. ROBERT H. SCHULLER

Thank You, God, for Today!

WHY DO I HAVE a rash on my chest?

What is that coming out of my surgical scar?

Why am I having breast pain?

What is going on with me?

Although I was at peace with my decision to forgo chemotherapy, I struggled to move forward with life. Another unsettling question floated around in my head, "Am I going to have a recurrence like my Aunt Addie?" I couldn't stop thinking that the cancer was more likely to come back in the first two to three years. Those statistics frightened me. But there was good news: oncologists tell patients that the risk of recurrence is highest in the first five years. And, if a patient makes it to five years, she has a good chance of remaining disease-free long term.

After a breast cancer patient completes her treatments, she transitions into survivorship mode. This may include meeting with a nutritionist, therapist, or attending a support group. For me, the first step was counseling. My goodness, I was an emotional wreck. Early one morning, I drove myself to see a psychiatrist who works with breast cancer patients.

"If I have to return to work now, I may quit my job because I am stressed out and sad," I told Dr. Berringer.

"Ms. Bass, with a mature mind, that most likely won't happen," the psychiatrist replied.

I spent the next half hour describing how the following traumatic events had left me sad: my recent triple-negative breast cancer diagnosis, a bilateral mastectomy, a surgery for a hematoma that I caused, the death of my aunt, and feelings of abandonment because my caregivers were gone.

"And my boss doesn't like me. Please, doctor, I don't want to return to work right now. I need more time off."

To my surprise, Dr. Berringer replied, "Although you may be clinically depressed, you appear to be unusually resilient. Also, Ms. Bass, I don't write medical excuses on first visits."

I thought, "What kind of insensitive and crazy response is that? Really?" It took every piece of restraint inside me to keep from falling onto the floor and begging the psychiatrist to write me a medical excuse. Now, wouldn't THAT have been immature and weird behavior for an adult? I wasn't ready to go back to work.

Eventually, I realized that I wasn't going to get any compassion or assistance from the psychiatrist. I should not have told her how I had overcome so much tragedy in the past: losing my mom, father, two brothers, favorite uncle, and my aunt. Sigh. I needed a medical excuse, not a medal for emotional resiliency. On the way home, I boohooed and wiped my runny nose like a 5-year-old. I was disappointed and angry that the psychiatrist had not written me a medical excuse to extend my leave.

Returning to work is easy when you feel valued and/or have a great boss. Although I had great coworkers, the controller who recruited me had recently retired. The new controller appeared to have a smirk on his face when I told him I had to leave for an unforeseen medical emergency, so I didn't feel valued. Sadly, I dreaded returning to my job in my emotional state, so I contemplated finding another psychiatrist to extend my medical leave. I was in a dark place.

A few days later, my son came home from camp and asked, "Mom, did you bathe today? You don't smell feminine, Mom, and your hair doesn't smell like other girls."

To avoid answering his question, I replied, "Christopher, hair is all you better be smelling."

My girls were gone; I didn't feel the same, so I didn't bathe every day. My son's observations were a wake-up call. I immediately realized that the psychiatrist had done me a *huge favor* by not extending my medical leave.

Truth be told, I was sad and worried about my cancer recurring. In fact, I didn't like to bathe because I didn't want to look at my surgical scars. Was I suffering from body-image sadness? All I wanted to do was sit around, Google triple-negative breast cancer, and watch Ellen at 4 p.m. Ellen made me laugh, and the show took my mind off my fear and sadness, and the fact that I hadn't bathed all day.

Hypocrisy is real. How could I repeat the late and great Dr. Robert Schuller's quote, "Tough times never last, but tough people do," to anyone who would listen, if they were experiencing a challenge, and yet not follow my own advice?

After my son's embarrassing observations, I realized that I had to *push through the pain* and make sure I took a shower every morning. How could I constantly remind Christopher about the importance of personal hygiene (Have you ever smelled the funk of a teenage boy after marching band practice? Rancid.), and sit around the house all day without taking a shower? Rancid.

Furthermore, it was time to be strong and make a paradigm shift to survival mode. I had to do it for Christopher until I was strong enough to realize I had to live for myself. There were moments when I experienced hopelessness, loneliness, and despair. My son was my lifeline.

The pre-cancer Ms. Bass was resilient and a victor instead of a victim, so I needed to go back to work and resume moving forward with my life. It was painfully difficult. So, I focused on the following scriptures.

"Men ought to always pray, and not to faint."
(KJV: LUKE 18:1)

"For God has not given us the spirit of fear,
but of power, and of love, and a sound mind."
(KJV: 2 TIMOTHY 1:7)

Then I read affirmations from, *Faith In The Valley*, by Iyanla
Vanzant. The following affirmation resonated with me:

"You know everything will turn out just fine. Even if it doesn't
feel like it right now, you know, This too shall pass."

I felt empowered: *kind of*. It was an arduous process.

A WEEK BEFORE I had to return to work, I spent my time
researching how I was going to strengthen my body's natural
defenses against cancer. The book *Anticancer, A New Way of
Life* by David Servan-Schreiber, MD, PhD, was very helpful. I
was fascinated with the author, who lived with brain cancer for
10 years. The book inspired me to take a deeper dive into understanding what foods feed and fight cancer. There are so many
diets: Gerson, Mediterranean, vegetarian, vegan, paleo, keto,
and macrobiotic. Dr. Servan-Schreiber seemed to favor a Mediterranean diet. Also, my oncologist recommended a Mediterranean
diet if I couldn't be a vegan. When I tried to be a vegan, I lost
too much weight, looked scrawny, and experienced dizzy spells.
Nevertheless, I have a lot of vegan friends, and they are healthy
and look great.

To get advice on how to increase my body's natural defense
system against cancer, I sought out help from an integrative
doctor. He was concerned about my anxiety, so he recommended
stress reduction techniques like exercise, yoga, and acupuncture.

Eventually, I developed a survival plan that includes eating
a plant-based diet, fruits, and whole grains. Also, I get acupuncture treatments for anxiety. This plan isn't too different from my

MARQUITA BASS

pre-cancer lifestyle. A person should gravitate toward a healthy diet that is pragmatic for her so she will stick with it. Now, about 10% of the time, I eat whatever I want (within reason). You can't stop living; however, keep in mind that food can either contribute to good health or kill you, but you can't stress over your diet.

Also, I make sure I maintain adequate vitamin D levels, greater than 50ng/mL, by taking a daily D3 supplement. It is important that you have your vitamin D level checked even if you have not been diagnosed with breast cancer. Dr. Margaret I. Cuomo, MD writes in her book, *A World Without Cancer*, "Compelling scientific research has persuaded me that vitamin D is a valuable cancer-preventing agent, and I would like to see government and the medical community do more to promote its benefits."

Fortunately, I was taking a supplement when I was diagnosed so my vitamin D level was slightly above 30ng/mL, which is considered acceptable. However, the integrative doctor I visited recommended levels between 50 and 70ng/mL for breast cancer survivors. Please be careful because there is such a thing as vitamin D toxicity. Therefore, I get my levels checked when I have a physical.

Furthermore, I focus on maintaining good selenium levels by eating two Brazil nuts a few days a week to avoid getting too much selenium. My oncologist is not a proponent of taking supplements other than vitamin D, so I focus on getting my nutrients in my diet. According to breastcancer.org, selenium may decrease the risk for prostate, colon, gastrointestinal, lung, and breast cancers. Selenium acts as an antioxidant.[1]

In order to overcome the sad feelings, I continued to pray. Fortunately, I found a support group for TNBC survivors. Unfortunately, most cities only have support groups for hormone-positive breast cancer patients.

The support group gave me the opportunity to share my

story with other cancer survivors who could relate to my fear. Many breast cancer survivors worry about their cancer coming back, especially TNBC patients, because every single research article highlights that triple-negative breast cancer is a disease with a poorer prognosis.

I met a wonderful lady named Mary at my first support group meeting. She was feisty, brilliant, and fearless. Also, she had started the support group. We dominated the meeting with our questions, input, and strong personalities. We had an instant connection, so we exchanged phone numbers. During a five-year friendship, we discovered that we had a lot in common. We attended Emory University at different times, shared similar personalities, followed politics, and enjoyed walking outdoors. Mary and I became confidantes, and we talked on the phone for hours about breast cancer, traumatic personal life experiences, our families, careers, our cats, guns, and orchids.

Mary taught me that there are more species of orchids than other plants. It was my pleasure to take my friend to a luncheon at the Atlanta Botanical Garden, where she was honored as a long-time volunteer in the orchid nursery. When Mary introduced me as her friend who was also a TNBC survivor, I felt honored and a sense of solidarity. Therefore, it didn't bother me when she shared my personal health information; we shared the journey and she was a motherly figure.

On the other hand, I had become irate a week earlier when another friend introduced me during lunch by saying, "This is my friend I told you was treated for an aggressive form of breast cancer." I was shocked and mortified, so I immediately excused myself from the table and left the restaurant before placing an order. I thought, "When did I become defined by my cancer?" Fuming, I sat in my car and cried as I fired off a text message to my friend that read, *"Why did you think that introduction was okay? You didn't have the right to share my medical history, in my presence, without my permission."* She immediately apologized.

I know cancer survivors who wear their disease on their sleeve and openly discuss their journey. That is their choice and great. Conversely, I know women like myself who chose to keep their journey private (until I wrote this book), and that personal choice is fine. My point here: please don't discuss another woman's breast cancer diagnosis or any illness and reveal her name without her consent.

Please be cautious, this is the time to make sure your internal *sensitivity chip* is not malfunctioning. Some breast cancer patients are hyper-sensitive and scared. Therefore, we don't want to hear stories about your friend, a friend of a friend, or family member who has died from breast cancer. We definitely don't care to listen to stories about a person who has metastatic disease while we are in the throes of our cancer battle.

ONE THURSDAY MORNING IN July of 2016, Mary called me, and in a cracking voice over the phone, she said, "Marquita, my cancer is back, and I have chronic lymphocytic leukemia."

Immediately I replied, *"I will call you back."* She probably thought, "I am devastated and all you can say is I will call you back." The news was too devastating for me to handle, and I didn't want to upset my friend by having a meltdown on the phone. So, I rushed to end the call. After I calmed down, I called her back the next day. We talked for hours about the recurrence and her plans to start chemotherapy.

Where had this meteor, cancer recurrence, come from unex-pectedly? I was tired of bad news. Her diagnosis was a shock, and my world began to crumble. I was afraid that Mary was going to die soon. Furthermore, I started to fear that my cancer was going to recur. I thought I had made progress because it had been four years since I was diagnosed. In reality, I was treading water in the middle of an ocean.

Mary had passed the 5-year-TNBC recurrence milestone. She was healthy, exercised consistently, followed the conventional treatment options, and was white. According to several studies, white women tend to have a more favorable outcome when it comes to any breast cancer diagnosis. More confusing for me, Mary had taken all the standard TNBC treatments. She had a mastectomy, radiation, and chemotherapy.

My good friend's cancer journey was complicated by the fact that she was treated for hormone-positive breast cancer in 1997. Therefore, she wasn't sure if the 2016 recurrence was in fact TNBC or a recurrence of her original hormone-positive cancer. TN typically recurs in the lungs, liver, and brain, and Mary had bone metastasis.

Out of the blue, Mary was diagnosed in 2011 with a new primary tumor in the other breast that was triple-negative breast cancer (hormone-receptor-negative). My goodness, the freaking new tumor had a new personality or biology. What the heck? This exact scenario happened to my neighbor, Valerie.

How does a patient start with hormone-receptor-positive cancer and end up with hormone-receptor-negative cancer? According to breastcancer.org, "Research has shown that the "personality" of the cancer may change when breast cancer comes back. For example, the hormone-receptor status may change from hormone-receptor-positive to hormone-receptor-negative."[2]

The last time I saw Mary alive was at the hospital a year after her 2016 recurrence. Her last words to me as I was leaving, choking back tears, were "Marquita, you have to write a book and tell the world that it is taking too long to find a targeted treatment for triple-negative breast cancer … women are dying. TNBC patients need the same type of treatment options that are available for other types of breast cancers. Also, you have to share the story about your orange hands." I turned around, took a deep breath, and looked at my friend in her frail face. Her face had a bright orange tone as if she had jaundice. I think cancer had spread to her liver.

"I will write my book and share my experience about my orange hands," I promised Mary. We laughed as we always did about my orange hands. I said, "See you later," which was rhetorical because I had a horrible feeling in the pit of my stomach that her death was near. From the sad look on her face, she also knew that death was imminent. To this day, I regret that I didn't run back and squeeze her tight and say, "Goodbye." Those words were too painful to say, and the pain and sadness I was experiencing were unbearable. I wanted to run out of her room and scream, "Why is another person I love dying from breast cancer?" It was a lot to handle. We said goodbye with our sad and loving glances into each other's eyes. Mary died the following day on July 3, 2017. I loved her.

Remember that I said breast cancer tragedies kept showing up in my life like an unwanted dinner guest? Well, two days before Mary died, a friend informed me that his daughter-in-law had died from hormone-receptor-positive breast cancer. My heart was sad for him and his wonderful family. It was difficult for me to fight the unwelcomed surges of the deep sadness I was experiencing after having two people die from breast cancer within a week.

ANOTHER IMPORTANT FACET OF survivorship includes surveillance. For me, it consisted of quarterly oncologist visits for blood work and a physical exam. Today, I visit the oncologist/my primary care doctor annually for cancer surveillance. During my first or second quarterly visit with Dr. Danbowski, he asked, "How much carrot juice are you drinking?"

"What do you mean?" I replied.

Dr. Danbowski raised my hands up toward my face and said, "Your palms are orange." He was right: the palms of my hands were orange. My niece, Tomika, and I looked at each other and laughed. We had not noticed my orange hands.

My goal was to drink a quart a day because carrot juice has anti-cancer properties. I added one cup to my morning smoothie. Then, I drank another cup as a morning and afternoon snack, followed by a final cup before bed. The oncologist cautioned me about the risks of getting too much beta-carotene from drinking too much carrot juice. Instead of drinking a quart of carrot juice a day, I reduced the amount to one cup. It took a while for my orange palms to turn back to pink.

WHEN I RETURNED TO work in August, I felt strong and determined to return to my life. I had my wellness plan, my cancer support group, and my faith. Still, I struggled to manage the fear of a cancer recurrence. The thoughts of a recurrence dominated my mind, so I worked long hours to take my mind off it.

Christopher made the snare line in the marching band, which was a big deal for a high school freshman. Guess what? I volunteered to work with the uniform committee. The old Ms. Bass was back. She was notorious for volunteering and over-committing herself. What was I thinking? As it turned out, I couldn't lift the heavy band uniforms without feeling pain. When I explained to the nice ladies that I had a recent mastectomy, they told me to sit down and sort gloves.

I guess I wasn't busy enough. Project management is one of my professional passions, so I was an adjunct project management instructor at a local university. When the administrator asked me to teach a class in October to cover for another professor, I agreed. This was two months after I had returned to work. Although I was busy at work and volunteering with the band, teaching was another opportunity to stay busy to keep my mind off cancer. I don't know where I found the energy to do everything I had going on.

Christopher lived with his dad every other week, so that

gave me a weekly break from parenting. Still, I was always tired. My body was healing from having two surgeries in six months. Nevertheless, if I had not been busy and overcommitted, I don't know what would have happened with my mental health. The fear of a cancer recurrence can be overwhelming and debilitating, so I had to keep moving.

One day, I had excruciating chest pain after I had eaten a lunch that was not on my healthy meal plan. As I drove home with Christopher after work, I repeated over and over like a mad woman, "This has to be a cancer recurrence, I am in so much pain in my chest. Oh my God."

I almost drove to the emergency room until I noticed my son's face. He looked scared, and his eyes were watery. Instead of going to the emergency room, I drove home, crawled into the bed, and cried. I didn't ask my son about school, homework, band practice, or his day. And I am not sure if he had dinner that night. On the way to school the next morning, Chris asked, "Mom, are you about to die?"

"I don't know, Son," I replied.

THREE YEARS BEFORE MY cancer surgery, I had been diagnosed with ovarian cysts. I worried that those cysts might turn into cancer. Therefore, I had a total hysterectomy in December 2012. This was six months after my bilateral mastectomy. Deep sadness tried to show its ugly face after my hysterectomy until I experienced several life-altering events. First, I watched a video of Gabby Gifford singing the national anthem after she was shot through the head. The Democratic Congresswoman from Arizona had survived an assassination attempt. I was astounded at her resilience, and my mood improved. If Congresswoman Gifford could emerge as a winner after being shot in the head, I could change my attitude about breast cancer and a hysterectomy.

Second, Pakistani activist Malala Yousafzai survived being shot by the Taliban in an assassination attempt because she had publicly advocated that girls should be allowed to go to school. Her survival was astounding, and later earned her a Nobel Peace Prize. She motivated me to do my best to move on and not succumb to sadness. Then, I found a blog, *Positives About Negatives*, written by Patricia Prijatel, the author of *Surviving Triple-Negative Breast Cancer*. Her advice: "Live every day as if the cancer isn't going to return."

One last memorable event that helped me to overcome deep sadness was when I heard my son play his tenor saxophone. He was auditioning for the Georgia All-State Band.

One evening while Christopher was practicing for his audition, I said, "Son, you sound great and I am excited and proud that you have made it to the final round. I think you can make the All-State Band this year." What I really meant was: "Son, you **NEED** to make the All-State Band *this year*—I may die soon. I want to travel to Savannah, Georgia, for the concert because it may be my last opportunity to go."

Because I was recuperating, I wasn't able to travel for three hours with Jerome and Christopher when he auditioned. As soon as Christopher walked into the audition room to play, I got a surprise call from Jerome. He said, "Listen," and placed the phone against the door so I could hear our son play. I was filled with joy and pride. The sound of Christopher playing was healing as I listened to him play every scale without hesitation. And, his sight-reading test sounded flawless.

At that moment, with tears pouring out of my eyes like water running from a faucet, I vowed to continue to fight and push through my sadness. I wanted to be a good mom, so I needed to be emotionally available to address my son's needs.

Fortunately, I could emerge from deep sadness quickly without it progressing to a point where I had to take medication for depression. It was always situational, and I got through the tough times. Who wouldn't experience deep sadness or depression after everything I had gone through, including the drastic body changes? According to breastcancer.org, "Depression is more than just feeling down in the dumps or sad for a few days. Sometimes, feelings of depression don't go away and can interfere with your everyday life."

Symptoms of depression can include:
• Sadness
• Loss of interest or pleasure in activities you used to enjoy
• Change in weight
• Difficulty sleeping or sleeping all the time
• Energy loss
• Feeling worthless, helpless, or hopeless
• Thoughts of death or suicide[3]

If you experience the symptoms mentioned above for more than two weeks; please seek professional help, immediately. This is not the time to be a superwoman.

Christopher made first chair in the All-State Band, so Jerome and I traveled to Savannah, Georgia, for the spring concerts. I was proud and happy.

PRAISE GOD! I HAVE been cancer-free for seven years. Every morning when I open my eyes, I say, "Thank You, God, for my good health today." I adhere to the message in Eckhart Tolle's book, *The Power of Now* – Live in the Presence. This spiritual teacher and author suggests that "By living aligned with the present moment, you also align your will with the Universal will." I am living so in the Present.

As I stated previously, most research shows that the recurrence rate for TNBC declines after five years. Conversely, hormone-positive cancers have a better outlook in the short-term, but these cancers can sometimes come back many years after treatments.[4,5] In Dr. Funk's book *Breasts: The Owner's Manual*, she tells triple-negative patients who make it to five years to "definitely pop open the champagne." Although I live in the Present, I am hyper-sensitive to any physical ailment I have. When I get sick, the first question I have is, "Has the cancer returned?"

In a study published in the *British Journal of Cancer,* the authors looked at a cohort of 873 TNBC patients from MD Anderson Breast Cancer Management System database (patients seen at the breast center or survivorship clinic between January 1, 1997 and April 7, 2015). The patients were at least five years from diagnosis with a median follow-up of 8.3 years. They concluded that, "the 10-year DRFS (distant relapse-free survival) was 92% and the 15-year DRFS was 84%."[6] These survival rates are excellent and encouraging. After I carefully reviewed the patient demographics, I noticed that 16% of the patients are black, and 67% are white, and the remaining patients are other races. I understand that there are study variables and limitations, that I am not aware of, that may be factored in the percentages. However, it seems like the survival rate for African Americans is disproportionately lower. Therefore, Dr. Funk, I will leave my Dom Perignon on ice for a few more years.

CHAPTER 9

The Diary of an Angry Black Woman
~ MARQUITA BASS

We Need Targeted Treatments for TNBC!

Dear Diary,

Why is there a disparity in death rates for all breast cancer types for African-American (AA) women compared to white women?

African-American women have a 42% higher breast cancer death rate compared to white women despite recent advancements in management of the disease.[1] Furthermore, a higher percentage of AA women are diagnosed with late-stage disease, compared to white women, and fewer AA women have smaller (<2 cm) tumors.[2,3]

The reasons for the disparities are vast. They may include socioeconomic and health factors. In a newspaper article, *Breast cancer is the most imperative health issue facing African American women*, Ricki Fairley, Vice President, Sisters Network, Inc., lists the following factors as reasons for the disparities.

1. Black women are not taking action. While 92% of black women agree breast health is important, only 25% have recently discussed breast health with their family, friends, or colleagues. And, only 17% have taken steps to understand their risk for breast cancer.
2. Black women lack information about the severity of breast cancer, breast cancer symptoms and the need for screening.

3. Black women take care of others at the expense of their own health.
4. Black Women are often at a more advanced stage upon detection.
5. Black women may not have access to health care or health insurance, so they may have lower frequency of and longer intervals between mammograms. This is because they may not have health insurance.
6. Black women may not follow up on abnormal mammogram results because they can't afford the diagnostic testing.
7. Black women often don't have access to the same prompt high quality treatment that white women have. They express that they are often feel disrespected by physicians and staff.
8. Black women face logistical barriers to accessing care (such as transportation issues or not being able to miss work or arrange for child care).
9. Black women fear a cancer diagnosis.[4]

More alarming, AA women are more likely to be diagnosed with aggressive cancers like triple-negative breast cancer (TNBC), and die from it. This is a tragic reality that has been verified and validated in study after study. I am amazed by the number of studies that have rendered the same dismal conclusion about the plight of African-American women and TNBC. My goal is to try to come up with solutions to close the health disparity gap. Also, I encourage AA women, especially younger women, to pay close attention to their breast health.

I would be remiss if I didn't mention that East Indian, Hispanic, and Ashkenazi Jewish women (due to BRCA1 mutations) also have disproportionately higher rates of triple-negative breast cancer. Jennifer Pietenpol, Ph.D., Director of the Vanderbilt-Ingram Cancer Center, called TNBC, "A pretty significant health problem from the standpoint that 11 percent of Caucasians, 17 percent of Hispanics, and 25 percent of African Americans have this type of breast cancer."[5] Her comments came in the article, *Different subtypes of triple-negative breast cancer respond to different therapies.*

Why does triple-negative breast cancer typically affect younger women?

In 2018, I attended a breast cancer conference in Philadelphia sponsored by Living Beyond Breast Cancer (lbbc.org). The organization's mission is to "work with women who have been diagnosed with breast cancer and their caregivers throughout their experience of diagnosis, treatment and recovery." LBBC is an organization that I relied upon for information on triple-negative breast cancer during the early years after my diagnosis.

At the conference, I met several younger women of different races and ethnicities with TNBC in their early 30s. They were healthy, vibrant, and ready to "keep it moving" despite their cancer diagnosis. One energetic woman from Texas pulled up her top unexpectedly during of our conversation in a crowded room, flashing her reconstructed boobs up close in my face. All I could say was, "Thank you for sharing." We both laughed uncontrollably.

According to the Young Survival Coalition, a group dedicated to young adults affected by breast cancer, "Although breast cancer in young women is rare, more than 250,000 women living in the United States today were diagnosed with it under age 40. In young women, breast cancer tends to be diagnosed in its later stages and be more aggressive. Young women also have a higher mortality rate and higher risk of metastatic recurrence (return of breast cancer in areas beyond the breast)."

What the heck! This is a description of classic triple-negative breast cancer. Furthermore, the following statistics from youngsurvival.org are unsettling.

Breast Cancer is Different in Younger Women
- There is no effective breast cancer screening tool yet for women under 40, most of whom have dense breast tissue that prevents routine mammograms from being a useful screening tool.
- Every year, more than 1,000 women under age 40 die from breast cancer.
- Nearly 80% of young women diagnosed with breast cancer find their breast abnormality themselves.
- The incidence of metastatic breast cancer at the time of initial diagnosis is apparently rising in women under the age of 40.

In addition, studies have shown that young African-American women face even greater challenges according to youngsurvival.org.
- African-American women under age 35 have rates of breast cancer two times higher than Caucasian women under age 35.
- African-American women under age 35 die from breast cancer three times as often as Caucasian women of the same age.

To complicate matters, younger women are too busy to "think about their breast health and cancer risk factors before they pink." They are on social media 24/7 or swiping left and right on their phones to find a date or the right hookup. They are getting boob jobs (warning: implants may make it harder to detect breast cancer when younger women start getting mammograms) and fat injected into their butts and lips. They are living their lives as phenomenal women while pursuing careers as entrepreneurs, educators, physicians, entertainers, corporate executives; and the list goes on. They are doing what they want to do, which is fantastic! Believe me, breast cancer is typically not on their radars.

However, "having breasts" is the **Number 1** risk factor for getting breast cancer. Moreover, according to researchers at the Centers for Disease Control and Prevention, "About 11% of all new cases of breast cancer in the United States are found in women younger than 45 years of age." Therefore, I wish more young ladies would take the time to learn about the deadly disease and their individual risk factors. *Younger women please pay attention to your breast health.*

A risk factor that may play a role in why younger women get TNBC breast cancer is the BRCA mutated gene. Several reputable studies have linked BRCA mutations to triple-negative breast cancer. In a Duke University genetic study published in the October 2013 issue of *Annals of Surgical Oncology*, the authors concluded that 43.8% of a total of 469 BRCA patients with TNBC were younger than 40 years old.[6] This is unfortunate because most women are not referred for genetic testing until they are diagnosed with breast cancer. Whereas if younger women were tested as a preventive measure, they could decide if they want to implement measures to avoid the deadly disease. Genetic testing is important even though only five to 10% of breast cancers are related to inherited mutations.

Thanks to a 2013 Supreme Court ruling that made genes accessible for commercial genetic testing, you can get BRCA testing from companies that specialize in genetic testing. Some commercially available gene analysis tests include a panel of genes ranging from 20 to 50 gene mutations. Baylor Genetics (baylorgenetics.com) was cited in one webinar I attended as a resource for cancer genetic testing. Again, genetic testing can be a powerful tool. It allows an individual to consider cancer prevention options. Now, this is "thinking about your breast health and cancer risk factors, before you pink!"

After my 2012 diagnosis, I participated in a University of Washington study, *Genomic Analysis of Inherited Breast Cancer*, where I was tested for more than 40 gene mutations. Several studies have found that BRCA gene mutations are not the only risk factors for breast cancer. After I submitted blood in several vials, I was a *happy* black woman when I received the following genetic analysis test results.

> **Result and interpretation: No mutations clearly damaging to gene function were identified in BRCA1, BRCA2 (*although I already knew this because it was a requirement of the study*) or any other known breast cancer genes. Variants are categorized as damaging if they clearly damage the gene's protein product.**

Why does triple-negative breast cancer disproportionately affect African-American women?

My friend Mary and I used to attend breast cancer conferences regularly. We were angry and disappointed that TNBC is the only breast cancer without a targeted treatment, so we wanted to hear from the experts. In 2013, we went to the *Glenn Family Breast Center Research Symposium: Treatment Resistant Breast Cancer Conference* in Atlanta. The target audience was oncologists, pathologists, and other medical professionals. I don't know how my friend orchestrated our registrations, but there was a name tag waiting for me when I arrived. Mary was amazing!

I drove like a race car driver to the Marriott Hotel in Buckhead to make sure I didn't miss the keynote speaker, Dr. Lisa Newman. She is currently the Chief of Breast Surgery at New York-Presbyterian/Weill Cornell Medical Center. Her presentation focused on African Ancestry and High-Risk TNBC. It was an honor and privilege to hear Dr. Newman speak.

During her presentation, Dr. Newman said she noticed "parallels between breast cancer of African-American and sub-Saharan African women." The observation led her to ask the question: "Is African ancestry associated with a heritable marker for high-risk breast cancer subtypes?" Subsequently, she traveled to Ghana to investigate triple-negative breast cancer in sub-Saharan African women. Due to the colonial-era slave trade, these women share ancestry with African-American women. As it turned out, approximately 60 percent of Ghanaian women who have breast cancer have triple-negative breast cancer, according to Dr. Newman. She also believes that genetic factors may play a role in TNBC, and European women may have a *different* disease compared to African-American women.

Unfortunately, most African-American women are not aware of their risk of getting TNBC. My goal is to increase awareness of the disease in the AA community. Also, there is no way I can ignore the magnitude of the struggles of all women who have heard the dreadful words, "It's a cancer." All cancer news is horrifying, and I am not downplaying the seriousness of any cancers. A triple-negative breast cancer diagnosis is especially horrifying because it is the *only* breast cancer without a targeted treatment.

How much longer is it going to take to validate the TNBC subtypes and find targeted treatments? Should the focus be on identifying a patient's subtype before treatment to advance research?

TNBC has historically been treated as a single disease entity in targeted therapy trials, but advances in gene expression profiling and other molecular diagnostic techniques over the last decade have revealed considerable biologic heterogeneity among TNBCs, including subgroups with distinct, targetable aberrations.[7]

My take: TNBC is treated as one disease, but it is not one disease. The different subtypes seem to react to different treatments. Therefore, I believe there is an **URGENT** need to validate the distinct diseases and develop drugs that are effective for each molecular type. Thank goodness, a lot of women survive triple-negative breast cancer with the current standard of care. But, we need precision medicine for triple-negative breast cancer to saves more lives.

The fact that triple-negative breast cancer is treated as one disease and most clinical trials (Clinicaltrials.gov) approach it as one disease, gnaws at me like a ferocious dog decimating a bone. I believe that this could be one of the primary reasons that research hasn't resulted in targeted treatments in a clinical setting for early stage disease.

How can one find a treatment for tumors that are different if she doesn't know what disease she is trying to cure? I ask this question over and over in my mind. *This has to change!* Do you think it would be beneficial to know "what gas is fueling a specific triple-negative tumor, before starting treatment?" This is particularly disturbing for me as research study, after study, has shown that TNBC molecular subtypes respond differently to different therapeutic agents.

I hear you saying that "I don't understand how the research process works, it is complicated, and I am uninformed, misinformed, and clueless." These responses are probably accurate. Even so, we all have opinions about things, and my SWAGs (Stupid Wild-Ass Guesses) may not be scientifically based. Nevertheless, they are based on my interpretation of evidence-based research findings.

Triple-negative breast cancer is killing too many women, especially African-American women. We are dropping like flies from the deadly cancer. For close to two decades, researchers have been saying:

- Triple-negative breast cancer is a disease with a poor prognosis.
- It is an unmet medical need.
- We need to find targeted treatments for the different subtypes.

I am waiting for the day when cancer researchers say, *"TNBC is no longer treated as one disease in clinical settings because we have validated the subtypes, and there are targeted treatments for early stage disease based on subtypes. Finally, triple-negative breast cancer has a targeted treatment like the other breast cancer types."* I will perform multiple praise dances after this wonderful day!!

One can't discuss TNBC subtypes without referencing the vanguard 2011 research study, *Identification of human triple-negative breast cancer subtypes and preclinical models for selection of targeted therapies,* conducted by Dr. Brian D. Lehmann and colleagues. Dr. Lehmann is a Research Assistant Professor at Vanderbilt University Medical Center. This is the first study to identify six subtypes of TNBC. The authors say their data may be useful in biomarker selection, drug discovery, and clinical trial design that will enable alignment of TNBC patients to appropriate targeted therapies."[8] According to a Web of Science Core Collection query, the study has been cited over 1,868 times.

I have conducted my own analysis of a variety of research studies about TNBC subtypes. Please see Appendix C to read my detailed analysis. My only goal is to highlight the significant research that has been done on TNBC subtypes. I was thrilled to find so many different researchers who have either validated Lehmann's original subtypes or found minor differences between their subtypes and Lehmann's.

Despite evidence-based findings that the subtypes respond to different treatments, the National Comprehensive Cancer Network (NCCN) guidelines still recommends that early-stage TNBC be treated with chemotherapy, like it is one disease. Unfortunately, research, to date, has not resulted in the completion of clinical trials and FDA approval of targeted treatments, unless the disease has advanced or is metastatic. This is unfortunate for newly diagnosed TNBC patients.

Why is significant progress taking so long? Maybe because:

- New drugs have to go through vigorous FDA-mandated multiple clinical trials, and the process takes a long time?
- TNBC only makes up 10 to 20% of all breast cancer (depending on the study), so it hasn't received the same attention as hormone-positive breast cancer?
- TNBC disproportionately affects African-American women, one of the most marginalized groups of women in society, and no one cares? *My goodness! This can't be the reason,* because women of all races and ethnicities are also affected, and are dying.

Honestly, the reason there isn't a targeted treatment is not important. We need to fix the problem—*NOW.*

Hopefully, it will not take half a century to find a targeted treatment. According to the authors of the Department of Defense Breast Cancer Research Program report, *The Breast Cancer Landscape*, "Breast cancer is a global problem. Worldwide, breast cancer accounts for nearly a quarter of all cancers in women and it is estimated that 2.1 million women will be diagnosed with the disease in 2018. In the United States, in 2019, it is estimated that 331,530 women will be diagnosed with breast cancer. The chance of a woman being diagnosed with breast cancer during her lifetime has increased from about 1 in 11 in 1975 to 1 in 8 today."[9] Moreover, half a million women die in the world every year with breast cancer, of which 150,000 are estimated to be TNBC cases. This equates to 30% of all breast cancer deaths.[10] Triple-negative breast cancer is only 10 to 20% of all breast cancers. The fact that it equates to approximately 30% of all breast cancer deaths is freaking mind-blowing, *at least for me.*

A triple-negative diagnosis can be devastating and earth-shattering for most women. I have met women who have become paralyzed by fear and are willing to forgo treatments because everything you read says, "TNBC is a disease with a poor prognosis" and the only treatments are "poison, cut, burn, and poison some more" and the prognosis is still poor. This is unfortunate and insane for the women who don't survive!

Repeated studies suggest that a subset of patients have tumors that are androgen receptor (AR) positive, and the tumors may be chemo-resistant. Will future clinical studies lead to changes in how the disease for AR patients is treated in clinical practice for early stage disease?

In 2018, I met a wonderful lady named Melissa who is from Pennsylvania. She is a funny, thoughtful, and beautiful woman with hair like Julia Roberts, in the movie *Pretty Woman*. We have stayed in touch, and we talk or text often. Melissa has become like a sister from another mother. My heart is sad that we are a part of the TNBC sisterhood.

Melissa was diagnosed with Stage 1 TNBC in 2018, so she had a lumpectomy to remove the tumor. Instead of taking conventional chemotherapy, she traveled to Georgia to receive treatments from an integrative oncologist. He promised her low dose chemotherapy using insulin potentiation therapy (IPT). It affects the metabolism of cancer cells to make them sensitive to chemo, so a lower dose of chemotherapy can be administered. More significant, Melissa's chemo and treatment were supposed to be based on the molecular make-up of her tumor according to a Caris Life Sciences report. According to carislifesciencs.org, their platform is to "fulfill the promise of precision medicine and to facilitate a deeper understanding of the biology of cancer and other complex diseases."

Melissa and I sat outside for lunch on a beautiful sunny, fall day, because she couldn't tolerate the smell of food inside the restaurant and was nauseated from chemotherapy. I felt super excited when Melissa said her chemo treatment was specific to her cancer. It was targeted treatment! My friend was getting what I was in search of when I was diagnosed: precision medicine for the molecular make-up of my tumor. I thought, "Wow! Treatment options have improved since 2012."

According to the authors of the research article, *Androgen receptor positive triple-negative breast cancer: Clinicopathologic, prognostic, and predictive features,* "The combination of Androgen Receptor positive and the Epidermal Growth Factor Receptor (EGFR gene) negative represents the Luminal Androgen Receptor (LAR) molecular subtype, with the best prognosis and may benefit the most from anti-androgen therapies."[11] A few months after Melissa left Georgia, she shared her Caris Life Sciences report with me. The reported showed that her tumor was Androgen Receptor (AR) positive and EGFR (Epidermal Growth Factor Receptor) negative. EGFR is a gene that may influence how breast cancer responds to treatment.

Based on Caris' analysis of her tumor:
1. Bicalutamide, enzalutamide – androgen antagonists – are therapies with ***potential benefit,***
2. Doxorubicin and cisplatin – chemo drugs – are therapies with ***uncertain benefit.***

Melissa was heartbroken and felt betrayed when she realized the integrative oncologist opted to still administer docetaxel and cisplatin although these chemo drugs were listed as therapies with uncertain benefit on her Caris report. The oncologist also added another chemo drug to her treatment, cyclophosphamide. More disappointing and confusing, the oncologist did not discuss Melissa's tumor AR status with her while she was in treatment, or review the recommended therapies outlined in her Caris report.

"You are the one who told me my tumor is Androgen Receptor-positive according to my Caris report," she said to me. "I am so upset because the doctor should have discussed this with me while I was in Georgia. I trusted him. He should have given me the option to decide if I wanted to proceed with chemotherapy that was listed as an uncertain benefit for my tumor or any chemo. Studies have shown that AR tumors may be chemo-resistant."

So, Melissa asked the doctor how he decided on her treatment. He said her cancer was most likely fueled by male hormones, and the Caris report "had two therapies with potential benefit: bicalutamide and enzalutamide. Also, he said, "Both of these therapies target the androgen receptor (AR). These are not chemotherapy agents, but a class of drugs known as androgen receptor inhibitors. They are approved to treat prostate cancer in men. They are not typically used in women, and they are not amenable to IPT."

With a price tag of $30K for the oncologist's services and $4200 to rent a condo in Atlanta, did my dear spend a large sum of money for a treatment she didn't need? Another million-dollar question is, *"Why didn't the doctor have a conversation with Melissa about her TN subtype while she was in Georgia?"* A year later, Melissa found herself back at square one with either residual disease or a recurrence. The reasons why are indeterminate. However, could one contributing factor be that the LAR subtype is possibly chemo-resistant, which has been proven by several researchers? (See my analysis in Appendix C.)

Melissa's story is important because AR-positive tumors have consistently been validated as a TNBC subtype in various research studies. Lehmann and his colleagues identified the LAR (Luminal Androgen Receptor) subtype in 2011.[12] In 2018, the authors of *Androgen receptor positive triple-negative breast cancer: Clinicopathologic, prognostic, and predictive features*, stated, "Overexpression of the androgen receptor (AR) charac-

terizes a distinct molecular subset of triple negative breast carcinomas (TNBC)."[13]

I am intrigued by other research studies concerning the LAR
subtype. For example, the authors of the 2015 study, *Subtyping
of Triple-Negative Breast Cancer: Implications for Therapy*,
stated, "Despite the promise of targeted therapies, cytotoxic
chemotherapy remains the mainstay of treatment for patients
with TNBC. In particular, the LAR subtype is predicted to have
the least benefit from traditional cytotoxic chemotherapy."[14]

Dr. Ruth O'Regan is a knowledgeable and respected oncologist and researcher on the TNBC scene. She oversees clinical
research at the University of Wisconsin Carbone Cancer Center
(UWCCC). I was delighted to hear Dr. O'Regan speak twice
when she was on staff at Emory Winship Cancer Institute. She
co-authored a meta-analysis review paper, *The Role of Androgen
in Triple-Negative Breast Cancer*, which states, "further investigation to elucidate the prognostic implications of AR in TNBC
is required. Routine AR evaluation by immunohistochemistry
(IHC) in TNBC could provide further insight in this direction."[15]
By routine investigation, I assume the authors are saying, "AR
status of triple-negative breast cancer tumors may be of value in
routine pathology reports." More promising, it appears that the
LAR subtype may represent 10 to 20% of TNBC tumors (depending on the study). Thus, routinely testing for AR status in
pathology reports could be beneficial. All TNBC cancer patients
may not benefit from chemotherapy, *after all*.

In another review article, *Genetic Markers in Triple-Negative
Breast Cancer*, the authors stated, "The therapeutic value of
screening for AR positivity is that this is an easily detectable
marker than can identify subgroups of TNBC patients who will
derive minimal clinical benefit from standard chemotherapy.
AR-dependent TNBC patients could benefit from targeted
therapy based on AR antagonists alone or in combination with
other chemical agents."[16]

Although my friend Melissa has the LAR subtype, and many studies have found that it has a low pathological complete response rate to chemo, a second oncologist told her, "she couldn't sleep at night if she didn't recommend chemotherapy." Melissa and I had hoped for a different response during her consultation. However, we understand that the oncologist is doing her job by following protocol and the standard of care as specified by NCCN guidelines. The directive instructs oncologists to treat early stage TNBC as one disease, with chemotherapy. Is this unfortunate for patients who may have tumors that may be chemo-resistant?

Thankfully, I found two Androgen Receptor (early-stage disease) clinical studies on Clinicaltrial.gov, and there may be more. The studies are: *Feasibility Study of Adjuvant Enzalutamide for the Treatment of Early Stage AR(+) Triple-negative breast cancer (Phase 2)* and *Ribociclib and Bicalutamide in AR+ TNBC (Phase 1)*. I pray that the results from these and similar studies lead to a change in how AR-positive TN tumors are treated in a clinical setting. This is encouraging and promising.

Why are all the recent FDA-approved treatments restricted to advanced and/or metastatic TNBC disease?

As of June 11, 2019, the FDA has approved the following treatments for TNBC.

1. Early Stage Disease – Chemotherapy without any consideration given to tumor characteristics. This has always been the standard of care for triple-negative breast cancer.

2. In 2018, the PARP inhibitor olaparib (Lynparza) was approved by the FDA for the treatment of advanced breast cancers with BRCA mutations. While not exclusively for patients with TNBC, it provides a new treatment option for a subset of patients with TNBC.

For the life of me, I don't understand why patients with BRCA mutations are not given the PARP inhibitor olaparib for early stage disease instead of chemotherapy. Or, because chemo is the recommended treatment of choice, why aren't patients given olaparib with chemotherapy for early stage disease?

"OlympiAD is the first phase III study to show an advantage of a PARP inhibitor over standard of care chemotherapy in breast cancer patients with a BRCA mutation" according to principal investigator, Mark E. Robson, MD. Dr. Robson is the Clinic Director of the Clinical Genetics Service at Memorial Sloan Kettering Cancer Center. The median progression-free survival (PFS) was improved by 2.8 months with olaparib. The objective response rate (ORR) was 59.9% with olaparib versus 28.8% with chemotherapy.[17] More interesting, the authors stated in the study conclusion, "While there was no statistically significant improvement in OS (overall survival) with olaparib compared to chemotherapy TPC (treatment of physician choice), there was the possibility of meaningful overall survival benefit among patients who had not received chemotherapy for metastatic disease. Olaparib was generally well-tolerated, with no evidence of cumulative toxicity during extended exposure."[18] This is fantastic news, so here is another one of my SWAGs. Is it unreasonable to guess: Will a patient with early stage disease who hasn't received any chemotherapy be able to avoid metastatic disease if she is given olaparib as a single medication? Just a thought.

3. In 2019, the FDA approved a combination of the immunotherapy drug, Tecentriq (atezolizumab) and the chemotherapy drug, Abraxane (nab-paclitaxel) for PD-L1 positive unresectable local advanced or metastatic *TNBC*. PD-L1 are types of proteins found

on cells in your body. I have one last SWAG: Can patients have their tumors tested for PD-L1, or is there a blood test that could identify TNBC patients who would benefit from immunotherapy drugs before the disease advances? Just a thought.

On December 11, 2018, Dr. Lisa Carey, a member of the Triple Negative Breast Cancer Foundation Advisory Board, told members of the organization that "incremental progress matters" and "there are clear and wonderful advances happening" when it comes to TNBC.[20] This is awesome news. Incremental progress is good, even if the recent FDA-approved therapies are for locally advanced or metastatic disease.

During the same conversation, Dr. Carey also said, "We're not going to stop using chemo, but we are looking at innovative ways of using the tools we have." As I've already said, my goal is not to launch a scathing attack against chemotherapy. *It saves lives!* And I don't mean to suggest that oncologists are not doing a great job. *They save lives.* Oncologists follow NCCN guidelines that "document evidence-based, consensus-driven management to ensure that all patients receive preventive, diagnostic, treatment, and supportive services that are most likely to lead to optimal outcomes." (nccn.org)

On the other hand, the verdict is out when it comes to the integrity of the individuals at NCCN's member institutions who participate in "consensus-driven management" of cancer treatment. According to an article in The New York Times,

> *"Dr. Craig B. Thompson, the chief executive of Memorial Sloan Kettering Cancer Center, said Tuesday that he would resign his seats on the boards of drug maker Merck and another public company, the latest fallout from a widening institutional reckoning over relationships between cancer center leaders and for-profit health care companies."*[19]

This news is unfortunate and makes one question the motives of individuals at NCCN member institutions when they decide on treatment options oncologists should follow. Is there a pervasive unreported conflict-of-interest problem at other NCCN member institutions? How would we know?

Furthermore, I'm particularly alarmed when I read studies like *Chemoresistance Evolution in Triple-Negative Breast Cancer Delineated by Single-Cell Sequencing,* where researchers from several respected institutions, including MD Anderson Cancer Center conclude: "Triple-negative breast cancer is an aggressive subtype that frequently develops resistance to chemotherapy."[21] This is disturbing because chemotherapy is the standard of care for TNBC. Again, a lot of women survive with the current standard of care, but too many women don't have a favorable outcome. This seems to be particularly true for African-American women. I am repeating what is continuously stated in TNBC research studies.

FOR THE SAKE OF the lives of the thousands of women who have TNBC, and the women who will be diagnosed in the future, we need targeted treatments for triple-negative breast cancer. Oncologists need to stop treating it as one disease. A lot of women survive triple-negative breast cancer, but it is an unmet need for approximately 30 to 40% of patients (this percentage could be different, depending on the study). Stacy Moulder, M.D. is a professor of Breast Medical Oncology at MD Anderson. In the article, *ARTEMIS clinical trial offers triple-negative patients personalized therapy,* Dr. Moulder stated, "Over half of patients have a tumor that's insensitive to chemotherapy, which is manifested as residual disease identified at the time of surgery. And 50 to 60 percent of that population will experience a recurrence of their cancer within two to three years."[22]

I am encouraged about MD Anderson's clinical trial,

ARTEMIS: A Robust TNBC Evaluation fraMework to Improve Survival. "The goal of this clinical research study is to learn if the use of imaging response and molecular testing on tumors can improve response to treatment in patients with triple-negative breast cancer by guiding patients with chemotherapy-sensitive tumors to receive standard chemotherapy and chemotherapy-insensitive tumors to consider a clinical trial."[23] I pray that this study leads to precision medicine.

Oncotype and Mammaprint are tests that tell hormone-positive patients if they need chemo, based on the risk that a tumor will metastasize to other parts of the body. Dr. Kathy D. Miller, keynote speaker at the September 2018 LBBC conference said, "The introduction of these tests is the biggest advance in breast cancer in the last 10 years because approximately 70% of hormone-positive breast cancer patients don't have to take chemo." I am elated for hormone-positive breast cancer patients because some of them can avoid the toxicity of chemotherapy drugs. TNBC patients need similar tests, in addition to targeted therapies for the different subtypes.

And we don't have decades to wait.

Signed,
An Angry Black Woman

EPILOGUE

ON MAY 13, 2019, EXACTLY seven years—minus a month—from my June 13, 2012, breast surgery, I was at Emory University Hospital for another breast surgery.

"Hello Ms. Bass, what surgery are you having today?" asked Dr. Lasken.

With tears pouring from my eyes, I responded, "I want to remove both implants. I know you said that you can remove the scar tissue and leave my implants intact. But you don't know if it's scar tissue, and I am over this. The implants have served me for seven years, and now I am over it."

DURING THE SUMMER OF 2017, I endured serious bruising on my left side near my breast implant after I slipped on water on ceramic tile in my kitchen. To avoid hitting my head, which could have been life-threatening, I broke the fall with my left arm beneath my breast. That fall gave me breast pain for two years. Eventually, a radiologist saw something on an MRI scan of the area around my implant, but she wasn't able to ascertain what it was.

There were six women in my circle during this time with breast cancer: two with hormone-positive cancer and four with triple-negative breast cancer. Anytime a friend or family member is dealing with breast cancer, especially TNBC, my mind goes there; I think my cancer could return any day. Breast cancer is an insidious disease, and one doesn't know, nor can one predict when or if it will show up again.

To try to determine what was going on near my left implant, I consulted my plastic surgeon, Dr. Lasken. He told me the only way to know what was going on around my implant was to "go in," although he thought it was nothing. His view did not make me feel at ease. Immediately, I felt the same fear that had ripped through my brain after my initial "it's a cancer" news. What if my cancer had returned?

In 2012, I had guarded my emotions on the day of surgery; I was determined to control my emotions and not cry. This time around, as I waited for surgery, I cried and looked sad. Everyone, including the nurse, surgeon, radiologist, and surgical nurse, saw me cry and blow my nose like a toddler. The radiologist asked, "Do you have a cold?"

"No," I replied. "I am scared."

The nurse who helped me get dressed for surgery reminded me of actress and comedian Tiffany Haddish. She displayed a lot of energy and was hilarious. Also, she picked up on my fear and sadness when she walked into the room.

"Ms. Bass, how are you doing?" she asked, in a particularly vibrant tone.

"I am scared," I replied.

"You have to be positive, Ms. Bass. My patients can't be sad and scared. I am going to take good care of you. Being sad is not an option. You will do great."

Then she laughed and gave me a huge bright smile as she prepped me for surgery. Her smile and enthusiasm were contagious, so I laughed. Each time she checked on me, she told jokes about different topics. The nurse was gregarious and funny. She joked about eye lashes and handmade ointment she had made *especially* for me, which turned out to be Vaseline. We also laughed about things I can't write about. At one point, I laughed so hard and loud it made me forget about being scared and the possibility of having more cancer. *Thank you, Tiffany!*

IT TURNED OUT THAT the fall had in fact caused a lot of scar tissue around my implant. AND NO NEW CANCER!!! I was thrilled! However, I was very sad once I was at home recovering after I looked at how my body had changed as a result of cancer. I have transformed from wearing 32G Panache bras, to a size 34C, to whatever cup size I want to be. This reality pushed me into in a state of inertia. All I wanted to do was sit around and do nothing during my recovery.

My mood shifted after I watched Beyoncé's *Homecoming* performance on Netflix. She looked exhausted from rehearsing and taking care of her children, not long after having beautiful twins. During an interview, she said she didn't feel like herself and thought she would never be the same. I thought, "I feel the exact same way for other reasons, and I don't feel like finishing my book." However, Beyoncé rehearsed and prepared for the show like a warrior. Beyoncé's determination, dedication, and drive emanated through the television. I could feel it! Consequently, I decided to move beyond my emotional pain and be thankful for my blessings. The next day, I started writing again.

AS I MENTIONED PREVIOUSLY, approximately half a million women die in the world every year with breast cancer, of which 150,000 are estimated to be TNBC cases.[1] This equates to 30% of all breast cancer deaths. Moreover, some researchers contend that triple-negative breast cancer has a poor prognosis, probably because it is not one disease and there is no targeted treatment. I pray for a targeted treatment for each subtype. I am optimistic and hopeful for substantial advances in my lifetime. Also, I am excited that I have met other long-term TNBC survivors since my initial diagnosis in 2012. Triple-negative breast cancer patients should have FAITH and HOPE for a positive outcome.

My final thoughts are: I can *only* pray that,
• More women actively manage their breast cancer risk factors. See Appendix A for a list of breast cancer risk factors. I hear some of you saying, "Well, you were health conscious prior to

your diagnosis, and you said you were 'managing your risk factors.' But still, you ended up with breast cancer." I hear you. My response is: I still believe that some breast cancers can be avoided, especially if you test positive for breast cancer genes prior to a diagnosis and decide to take steps to reduce your chances of getting breast cancer. Furthermore, if you manage your risk factors, it may be particularly beneficial for preventing hormone-positive cancers, as female hormones seem to be major promoters of the tumors. Because the intricacies of the different subtypes of TNBC are still being studied and sorted out, it is hard to know what the main tumor promoters are. However, I have met several triple-negative breast cancer patients, including myself, who had traumatic and/or life altering experiences prior to their diagnosis, which I find interesting. Furthermore, some TNBCs seem to be driven by BRCA gene mutations, an overexpression of Androgen Receptor, and immune system malfunctions because some of the tumors have high levels of tumor infiltrating lymphocytes. A tumor-infiltrating lymphocyte (TIL) is an immune cell that has moved from the blood into a tumor to try and attack the cancer.[2] Interestingly, according to the authors of, *Heterogeneity of tumour-infiltrating lymphocytes in breast cancer and its prognostic significance*, "TILs were associated with outcome in TNBC patients, as well as having prognostic significance for recurrent tumours."[3]

- More women actively focus on early detection for all breast cancer types. The sooner one is diagnosed with any type of cancer, the better the outcome. Early detection could save your life. *It may have saved my life!*

- Women, young and old, can take advantage of genetic testing for *all* known breast cancer genes. Tests are commercially available. According to the authors of *The Management of Early Stage and Metastatic Triple-negative breast cancer: A Review,* "BRCA mutations are more common among those with TNBC (~20%) and may have therapeutic implications."[4]

- Patients may better understand that "Chemotherapy has certainly improved over the years, but with chemotherapy alone, the residual risk remains substantially higher, between 30% and 40%."[5] This means that "approximately 40% of patients with stage I-III triple-negative breast cancer (TNBC) recur after standard treatment, while the remaining 60% experience long-term disease-free survival (DFS)."[6] This is critical information because research has shown that each TNBC subtype has biologic differences that behave differently to therapeutic agents (see Appendix C) which may play a role in why some tumors do not respond to treatment. *Most patients survive TNBC, which is good news.*
- Women have access to the diagnostic tool that is best for their breast cancer risk factors. For instance, ultrasounds and/or MRI screenings may be more effective screenings tools for women with dense breasts. Several research studies have shown that dense breast tissue shows up as white images on mammograms; thus, it may be hard to see tumors. TNBC can be aggressive, and the prognosis is poor. So, it is imperative that it is diagnosed sooner rather than later. *Women need to advocate for themselves when it comes to getting the best screening test for their specific risk factors.*
- All women have access to quality health care, regardless of income. Most states have resources for women to get either free or affordable breast cancer screenings. A Google search will give you a list of organizations that assist women with paying for mammograms. Please don't allow your income to keep you from getting routine screenings.

AS FAR AS MY life now, I live every day, *as much as possible,* as if the cancer is not going to return. I would not be human if I didn't get spooked occasionally, especially if I feel sensation near my chest wall, feel a lump under my armpits, or get any type of bump or funny looking mole anywhere on my body. As I stated, since my diagnosis, I have met other women who have survived triple-negative breast cancer. I met a lovely lady at a conference who is a 19-year survivor. There is hope for TNBC patients. I give God the Glory that I have been cancer free for seven years. Still, I am treading water in the middle of the ocean, although the waves of the tsunami of my initial breast cancer diagnosis have calmed down. Thank goodness, I have learned how to relax and smell the roses. Health is Wealth, so I am focused on being emotionally, spiritually, and physically healthy. I still wake up every morning and say, "Thank You, God, for today."

Because I am inherently intellectually curious, I have gotten two advanced degrees since my son, Christopher, left for college in 2016. Finally, I am living for me and not for my child. Admittedly, it has been difficult to move forward with a life that is not focused on my son's world and activities. Yay! I am making progress.

One of my goals is to continue to follow TNBC research and to increase awareness of the disease. I am particularly intrigued by John Hopkin's mistletoe clinical trial for all types of cancers.[7] Hopefully, the results will be significant for breast cancer patients. I met a lady online who had surgery and took mistletoe injections for triple-negative breast cancer; she is a nine-year survivor. Please listen carefully: I am not encouraging or discouraging alternative treatments, just sharing information. I know women who have experienced good results with integrative, alternative and conventional therapies. According to cancer.gov:

- Mistletoe is a semiparasitic plant that has been used for centuries to treat numerous human ailments.
- Mistletoe is used commonly in Europe, where a variety of different extracts are manufactured and marketed as injectable prescription drugs. These injectable drugs are not available commercially in the United States and are not approved as a treatment for people with cancer.

- Mistletoe is one of the most widely studied Complementary and Alternative medicine (CAM) therapies for cancer. In certain European countries, the preparations made from European mistletoe (*Viscum album*, Loranthaceae) are among the most prescribed drugs offered to cancer patients.
- Although mistletoe plants and berries are considered poisonous to humans, few serious side effects have been associated with mistletoe extract use.
- The use of mistletoe as a treatment for people with cancer has been investigated in clinical studies. Reports of improved survival and/or quality of life have been common, but many of the studies had major weaknesses that raise doubts about the reliability of the findings.
- At present, the use of mistletoe cannot be recommended outside the context of well-designed clinical trials. Such trials will be valuable to determine more clearly whether mistletoe can be useful in the treatment of specific subsets of cancer patients.[8]

My son, Christopher, lives on the west coast. He left Berklee after one year to focus on his music aspirations. Jerome and I raised him to be fearless when it comes to following his dreams and aspirations. He didn't have any reservations about leaving the nest.

I didn't notice another woman's chest before my mastectomy. I was too busy trying to conceal my breasts, especially in a professional setting. I didn't like the attention. So, I wore suits to work, and I typically kept my jacket on. Today, I notice other women because I don't have breasts which could be some form of unconscious grief. I don't know.

My daily prayer is: *"God, how do I get my sexy back after such drastic body changes as I continue to take steps toward love and self-acceptance?"*

APPENDIX A

According to clevelandclinic.org
(https://my.clevelandclinic.org/health/diseases/3986-breast-cancer), breast cancer risk factors are either controllable or uncontrollable.

Controllable risk factors for breast cancer

- **Alcohol consumption.** The risk of breast cancer increases with the amount of alcohol consumed. For instance, women who consume 2 or 3 alcoholic beverages daily have an approximately 20 percent higher risk of getting breast cancer than women who do not drink at all.

- **Body weight.** Being obese is a risk factor for breast cancer. It is important to eat a healthy diet and exercise regularly.

- **Breast implants.** Having silicone breast implants and resulting scar tissue make it harder to distinguish problems on regular mammograms. It is best to have a few more images (called implant displacement views) to improve the examination.

- **Choosing not to breastfeed.** Not breastfeeding can raise the risk.

- **Using hormone-based prescriptions.** This includes using hormone replacement therapy during menopause for more than 5 years and taking certain types of birth control pills.

Non-controllable risk factors for breast cancer

- **Being a woman.** Although men do get breast cancer, it is far more common in women.

- **Breast density.** You are at higher risk of breast cancer if you have dense breasts. It can also make it harder to see tumors during mammograms.

- **Getting older.** Aging is a factor. A majority of new breast cancer diagnoses come after the age of 55.

- **Reproductive factors.** These include getting your period before age 12, entering menopause after age 55, having no children, or having your first child after 30.

- **Exposure to radiation.** This type of exposure could result from having many fluoroscopy X-rays or from being treated with radiation to the chest area.

- **Having a family history of breast cancer, or having genetic mutations related to certain types of breast cancer.** Family history that includes having a first degree relative (mother, sister, daughter, father, brother, son) with breast cancer poses a higher risk for you. If you have more than one relative on either side of your family with breast cancer, you have a higher risk. In terms of genetic mutations, these include changes to genes like BRCA1 and BRCA2.

- **Having already had breast cancer.** The risk is higher for you if you have already had breast cancer and/or certain types of benign breast conditions such as lobular carcinoma in situ, ductal carcinoma in situ, or atypical hyperplasia.

APPENDIX B

<u>Less Common Breast Cancer Types</u>

Each of these types of breast cancer occurs in fewer than 5% of all cases that are diagnosed.
(https://www.verywellhealth.com/invasive-infiltrating-breast-cancer-430612)

A. Metaplastic breast cancer: a rare form of breast cancer that is often treated aggressively and has uncertain prognosis.

B. Adenoid cystic carcinoma: named for their microscopic appearance, these cancer cells resemble glandular and cystic cells. Usually not aggressive, this type of breast cancer has a good chance of recovery after treatment.

C. Mixed tumors: Tumors that are composed of different types of cancer cells, such as invasive ductal and lobular, are referred to as mixed tumors.

D. Mucinous (colloid) carcinoma: quite rare, this type of breast cancer produces mucous but has a good prognosis after treatment.

E. Sarcomas of the breast: sarcomas are cancers that form in connective tissue. Most breast cancers are carcinomas, which form in epithelial tissue.

F. Angiosarcoma: this rare type of breast cancer starts in cells that line the blood vessels within your breast or underarm area. It can result from radiation treatments and is apt to grow and spread quickly.

G. Phyllodes tumor (cystosarcoma phyllodes): named for its leaf-shaped growth pattern, these tumors are often harmless. If they are cancerous, surgery is required; Phyllodes tumors will not benefit from chemotherapy or radiation treatments.

H. Tubular carcinoma: a rare type of breast cancer, it takes its name from its microscopic appearance and has a better prognosis than most forms of invasive breast cancer.

I. Paget's disease of the nipple: shows up in and around the nipple and usually signals the presence of breast cancer beneath the skin.

APPENDIX C

I have reviewed various research studies on triple-negative breast subtypes. Based on the experts cited in the table and figures below, there appears to be four or six TNBC subtypes. They have been validated by various studies.

Table 1

Date	Reference Title	Study Highlights
2011	*Identification of human triple-negative breast cancer subtypes and preclinical models for selection of targeted therapies*[1]	**Lehmann** study identified 6 Subtypes: 1. Basal-like 1**(BL1)** 2. Basal-like 2 **(BL2)** 3. Mesenchymal **M** 4. Mesenchymal Stem-Like **(MSL)** 5. Immunomodulatory **(IM)** 6. Luminal Androgen Receptor **(LAR)** "Analyzed gene expression (GE) profiles from 21 breast cancer data sets and identified **587 TNBC cases.**"
2012	*TNBC type: A Subtyping Tool for Triple-Negative Breast Cancer*[2]	**Lehmann** was a part of a Vanderbilt group that "offered a user-friendly web interface to predict the subtypes for new TNBC samples that may facilitate diagnostics, biomarker selection, drug discovery, and the more tailored treatment of breast cancer."
2013	*Differential response to neoadjuvant*	"We revalidated the **Lehmann** and Bauer et al. experiments

Date	Reference Title	Study Highlights
	chemotherapy among 7 triple-negative breast cancer molecular subtypes[3]	using files from public datasets. We applied these methods to **146 TNBC patients** with gene expression obtained from June 2000 to March 2010 at our institution." An Unstable subtype (**UNC**) was added.
2013	*Identification of Prognosis-Relevant Subgroups in Patients with Chemoresistant Triple-negative breast cancer*[4]	"We developed a **clinically relevant signature** for patients with chemoresistant TNBC. The TNBC subgroup predicted to have relatively favorable prognosis was characterized by high expression of 'luminal-like' genes (**androgen-receptor [AR]** and GATA3); while the subgroup with worse prognosis was characterized by expression of cancer stem-cell markers."
2014	*Triple-negative breast cancer subtypes and pathologic complete-response rate to neoadjuvant chemotherapy: Results from the GEICAM/2006-2003 study*[5]	Another research group suggests that **Lehmann** "TNBC subtypes can predict tumor response to neoadjuvant chemotherapy, supporting their potential clinical utility in diagnosis, treatment selection and drug development, bringing TNBC patients a step closer to personalized medicine." Cohort: **94 enrolled patients**

Date	Reference Title	Study Highlights
2015	*Subtyping of Triple-Negative Breast Cancer: Implications for Therapy*[6]	**Lehmann** and other researchers validated their subtyping by using TNBC RNA sequencing data from The Cancer Genome Analysis (TCGA). "We are translating our preclinical findings into targeted, subtype-specific clinical trials for patients with TNBC based on our understanding of the biologic drivers of the different TNBC subtypes. Despite the promise of targeted therapies, cytotoxic chemotherapy remains the mainstay of treatment for patients with TNBC. In particular, the LAR subtype is predicted to have the least benefit from traditional cytotoxic chemotherapy. This is problematic not only because of the numerous toxicities of cytotoxic chemotherapy but also because recurrence rates after early stage disease remain high, and the survival of patients who have metastatic disease remains dismal. We validated our subtyping by using TNBC RNA sequencing data from TCGA. We determined a statistically similar distribution of subtypes across **163 TNBC** cases from The Cancer Genomic Atlas (TCGA.)." **See Figure 1,** below details of therapeutic treatments by TNBC subtypes.

Date	Reference Title	Study Highlights
2015	*Role of the Androgen Receptor in Triple-Negative Breast Cancer*[7]	"AR identification has been a major advance in the treatment of TNBC tumors. AR represents a novel therapeutic target in TNBC, which has an otherwise inferior prognosis. Based on promising early clinical data, we anticipate that the newer, more potent antiandrogens will significantly improve outcomes and likely will be the first targeted therapy available for what to date has been an orphan disease."
2015	*Gene-expression molecular subtyping of triple-negative breast cancer tumours: Importance of immune response*[8]	"We identified three subtypes of triple-negative patients: **luminal androgen receptor** (22%), basal-like with low immune response and high M2-like macrophages (45%), and basal-enriched with high immune response and lowM2-like macrophages (33%)." **Patient Cohort = 87**
2016	Refinement of Triple-Negative Breast Cancer Molecular Subtypes: Implications for Neoadjuvant Chemotherapy Selection[9]	**Lehmann** and other researchers "provided significant evidence that the **IM** and **MSL** TNBC subtypes represent tumors with substantial infiltrating lymphocytes and tumor-associated mesenchymal cells, respectively, and led us to refine our original TNBCtype (**BL1, BL2, IM, M, MSL** and **LAR**) to TNBCtype-4 (**BL1, BL2, M** and **LAR**). In a retrospective

Date	Reference Title	Study Highlights
		analysis of gene expression datasets from five clinical trials we determined the predictive value of TNBCtype-4 subtypes in response to neoadjuvant chemotherapy."
2017	Triple-Negative Breast Cancer Next-Generation Sequencing for Target Identification[10]	"Analysis of the TNBC subtypes has shown differing clinical outcomes and varying responses to therapy, both in the neoadjuvant and postsurgical settings. These inherent differences related to TNBC subclassification have resulted in a renewed effort to identify driver mutations and more appropriate targeted treatment." **Figure 2** summarizes the molecular classification of TNBC and lists potential matched therapies.
2018	*Genetic Markers in Triple-Negative Breast Cancer*[11]	"In spite of intensive research into finding new molecular biomarkers and designing personalized therapeutic approaches, BRCA mutational status is the only clinically validated biomarker for personalized therapy in TNBC." **Figure 3** summarizes the molecular classification of TNBC and lists potential therapies.

Figure 1 – 2015/*Subtyping of Triple-Negative Breast Cancer:*
Implications for Therapy[6]

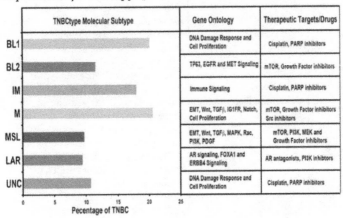

Figure 2 – *Triple-Negative Breast Cancer*
Next-Generation Sequencing for Target Identification[9]

TNBC Subtype	Genes Expressed	Potential Therapies
BL1	Cell cycle, DNA damage repair	PARP, Platinum
BL2	Growth Factor, Myoepithelial	PARP, Platinum
M	EMT, Growth Factor	Tyrosine kinase inhibitors, PI3K/mTOR inhibitors
MSL	EMT, Growth factor Proliferation (decreased)	Tyrosine kinase inhibitors, PI3K/mTOR inhibitors
IM	Immune signal	Anti-PD-L1 inhibitors
LAR	AR	AR targeted, PI3K inhibitors

Figure 3 – *Genetic Markers in Triple-Negative Breast Cancer*[11]

TNBC Subtype	Chemo Sensitivity	Potential Therapy
BL1	Very good	Cisplatin, PARP inhibitors
BL2	Very poor	Cisplatin; PARP and growth factor inhibitors
M	Medium	-
MSL	Medium	PI3K /mTOR, Src inibitors
IM	Medium	PI3K/mTOR, Src inibitors
LAR	Poor	AR antagonist; PI3K, Hsp90 inhibitors

REFERENCES

Chapter 1: "It's a Cancer"

1 Lawrence W. Bassett, MD, FACR, Karen Conner, and MS, IV., The Abnormal Mammogram, *Holland-Frei Cancer Medicine. 6th edition:* Retrieved from: https://www.ncbi.nlm.nih.gov/books/NBK12642/.

2 American Cancer Society, Breast Cancer Facts & Figures 2017-2018 (2017), accessed September 26, 2018, https://www.cancer.org/content/dam/cancer-org/research/cancer-facts-and-statistics/breast-cancer-facts-and-figures/breast-cancer-facts-and-figures-2017-2018.pdf.

3 Breastcancer.org, accessed September 26, 2018 from, https://www.breastcancer.org/symptoms/types/idc.

4 Breastcancer.org, accessed September 26, 2018 from, https://www.breastcancer.org/symptoms/types/ilc.

5 Breastcancer.org, accessed September 26, 2018 from, https://www.breastcancer.org/symptoms/types/inflammatory.

6 Breastcancer.org, accessed September 26, 2018 from, https://www.breastcancer.org/symptoms/types/ilc.

7 Breastcancer.org, accessed September 26, 2018 from, https://www.breastcancer.org/symptoms/types/ilc.

8 Ravdin, Peter M., Hormone Replacement Therapy and the Increase in the Incidence of Invasive Lobular Cancer, *Breast Disease*, vol. 30, no. 1, pp. 3-8, 2009. accessed September 26, 2018, from https://content.iospress.com/articles/breast-disease/bd000283.

9 Schneider, A. P., 2nd, Zainer, C. M., Kubat, C. K., Mullen, N. K., & Windisch, A. K. (2014). The breast cancer epidemic: 10 facts. *The Linacre Quarterly*, *81*(3), 244–277. doi:10.1179/2050854914Y.0000000027

10 Blows FM, Driver KE, Schmidt MK, et al. Subtyping of breast cancer by immunohistochemistry to investigate a relationship between subtype and short and long-survival: a collaborative analysis of data for 10,159 cases from 12 studies. *PLoS Med*. 2010;7: e1000279.

11 Haque R, Ahmed SA, Inzhakova G, et al. Impact of breast cancer subtypes and treatment on survival: an analysis spanning two decades. *Cancer Epidemiol Biomarkers Prev*. 2012;21: 1848-1855.

12 Bianchini G, Balko JM, Mayer IA, Sanders ME, Gianni L. Triple-negative breast cancer: challenges and opportunities of a heterogeneous disease. *Nature Rev Clin Oncol*. 2016;13: 674-690.

13 Cancer.gov, accessed on September 26, 2018 from, https://www.cancer.gov/types/metastatic-cancer.

Chapter 2: "Let the Curtain Go Up"

1 Kunihiko Itoh, Nobuhiro Maruchi, Breast Cancer In Patients With Hashimoto's Thyroiditis, *The Lancet*, Volume 306, Issue 7945, 6 December 1975, Pages 1119-1121.

Chapter 3: "Making Tough Decisions"

1. Eric C. Dietze, Christopher Sistrunk, Gustavo Miranda-Carboni, Ruth O'Regan, and Victoria L. Seewaldt, Triple-negative breast cancer in African-American women: disparities versus biology, Nat Rev Cancer. 2015 Apr; 15(4): 248–254.

2 Gábor Rubovszky, Zsolt Horváth, Recent Advances in the Neoadjuvant Treatment of Breast Cancer, *Journal of Breast Cancer*. 2017 Jun; 20(2): 119–131.

3 InformedHealth.org [Internet]. Cologne, Germany: Institute for Quality and Efficiency in Health Care (IQWiG); 2006-. Recurrent non-metastatic breast cancer. 2012 Sep 13 [Updated 2017 Jul 27]. Available from: https://www.ncbi.nlm.nih.gov/books/NBK279424/.

4 Breastcancer.org, accessed January 15, 2019 from, https://www.breastcancer.org/treatment/surgery/mast_vs_lump.

5 American Cancer Society, accessed January 15, 2019 from, https://www.cancer.org/latest-news/when-breast-cancer-comes-back.html.

6 Akshara Raghavendra, MD, Arup K. Sinha, Huong T. Le-Petross, MD, et al., Mammographic Breast Density Is Associated With the Development of Contralateral Breast Cancer, *Cancer* 2017;123:1935-40.

7 Akshara Raghavendra, MD, Arup K. Sinha, Huong T. Le-Petross, MD, et al., Mammographic Breast Density Is Associated With the Development of Contralateral Breast Cancer, *Cancer* 2017;123:1935-40.

8 Breastcancer.org, accessed January 15, 2019 from, https://www.cancer.org/cancer/breast-cancer/risk-and-prevention/breast-cancer-risk-factors-you-cannot-change.html.

9 Breastcancer.org, accessed July 2, 2019 from, https://www.breastcancer.org/treatment/surgery/reconstruction/finding-surgeon.

Chapter 4: Preparing for Surgery: Battlefield in My Mind

1 Kassam F, Enright K, Dent R, et al. Survival outcomes for patients with metastatic triple-negative breast cancer: implications for clinical practice and trial design. *Clinical Breast Cancer* 2009;9:29-33.

2 Joyce O'Shaughnessy, M.D., Cynthia Osborne, M.D., John E. Pippen, M.D., Mark Yoffe, M.D., Debra Patt, M.D., Christine Rocha, M.Sc., Ingrid Chou Koo, Ph.D., Barry M. Sherman, M.D., and Charles Bradley, Ph.D., Iniparib plus Chemotherapy in Metastatic Triple-Negative Breast Cancer, *The New England Journal of Medicine*, 2011; 364:205-214.

3 MDS-Foundation.org, accessed February 13, 2019 from, https://www.mds-foundation.org/what-is-mds.

Chapter 5: The Bipolar Patient

1 Breastcancer.org, accessed March 5, 2018 from,
https://www.breastcancer.org/tips/intimacy/loss_of_libido.

2 Cancer.gov, accessed March 5, 2018 from, https://www.cancer.org/treatment/treat-
ments-and-side-effects/physical-side-effects/fertility-and-sexual-side-effects/sexual-
ity-for-women-with-cancer/chemo.html.

3 Tousimis, E., & Haslinger, M. (2018). Overview of indications for nipple sparing
mastectomy. *Gland surgery, 7*(3), 288–300. doi:10.21037/gs.2017.11.11.

4 Cancer.gov, accessed March 5, 201 from, ttps://www.cancer.gov/about-cancer/diag-
nosis-staging/staging/sentinel-node-biopsy-fact-sheet.

Chapter 7: None of this Information Makes Sense to Me!

1 P. J, Westenend, C. J. C. Meurs, & R. A. M. Damhuis, Tumor size and vascular invasion predict distant metastasis in stage I breast cancer. Grade distinguishes early and
late metastasis. *J Clin Pathol* 2005;58:196–201.

2 William D. Foulkes, M.B., B.S., Ph.D., Ian E. Smith, M.D., and Jorge S. Reis-Filho,
M.D., Ph.D, Current Concepts: Triple-negative breast cancer, *N Engl J Med 2010*;
363:1938-1948.

3 Godwin JE et al, Neutropenia, *Medscape*, May 2011.

4 Lehmann BC, Bauer JA, Chen Xi, et al. Identification of human triple-negative
breast cancer subtypes and preclinical models for selection of targeted therapies, J
Clin Invest. 2011;121(7):2750-2767. https://doi.org/10.1172/JCI45014.
2011;121(7):2750-2767. https://doi.org/10.1172/JCI45014.

5 Lisa A. Carey, Directed Therapy of Subtypes of Triple-Negative Breast Cancer, *The
Oncologist* 2011 vol. 16 Supplement 1 71-78.

6 Stewart RL, Updike KL, Factor RE, et al, A multigene assay determines risk of recurrence in patients with triple-negative breast cancer, *Cancer Research*, May 2,
2019; DOI: 10.1158/0008-5472.CAN-18-3014.

7 L.A. Carey, E.C. Dees, L. Sawyer, L. Gatti, D.T. Moore, F. Collichio, et al., The
triple-negative paradox: primary tumor chemosensitivity of breast cancer subtypes,
Clin. Cancer Res. 13 (2007) 2329–2334, http://dx.doi.org/10.1158/1078-0432.

Chapter 8: Thank You, God, for Today

1 Breastcancer.org, accessed on May 19, 2019 from,
https://www.breastcancer.org/tips/nutrition/supplements/known/selenium.

2 Breastcancer.org, accessed on May 19, 2019 from,
https://www.breastcancer.org/symptoms/diagnosis/recurrent.

3 Breastcancer.org, accessed on May 19, 2019 from,
https://www.breastcancer.org/treatment/side_effects/depression Blows FM,

4 Haque R, Ahmed SA, Inzhakova G, et al., Impact of breast cancer subtypes and treatment on survival: an analysis spanning two decades. *Cancer Epidemiol Biomarkers Prev*. 2012;21: 1848-1855.

5 Blows FM, Driver KE, Schmidt MK, et al., Subtyping of breast cancer by immunohistochemistry to investigate a relationship between subtype and short and long-survival: a collaborative analysis of data for 10,159 cases from 12 studies. *PLoS Med*. 2010;7: e1000279.

6 Reddy SM, Barcenas CH, Sinha AK, et al., Long-term survival outcomes of triple receptor negative breast cancer survivors who are disease free at 5 years and relationship with low hormone receptor positivity, *British Journal of Cancer* (2018) 118, 17–23 | doi: 10.1038/bjc.2017.379.

Chapter 9: The Diary of an Angry Black Woman

1 Foy, K. C., Fisher, J. L., Lustberg, M. B., et al. Disparities in breast cancer tumor characteristics, treatment, time to treatment, and survival probability among African American and white women. *NPJ breast cancer*, *4*, 7. doi:10.1038/s41523-018-0059-5.

2 Kurian, A. W., Fish, K., Shema, S. J. & Clarke, C. A. Lifetime risks of specific breast cancer subtypes among women in four racial/ethnic groups. *Breast Cancer Res* 12, R99, https://doi.org/10.1186/bcr2780 (2010).

3 Daly, B. & Olopade, O. I. A perfect storm: How tumor biology, genomics, and health care delivery patterns collide to create a racial survival disparity in breast cancer and proposed interventions for change. *Cancer J. Clin*. 65, 221–238 (2015).

4 The Charleston Chronicle. *Breast cancer is the most imperative health issue facing African American women*. Accessed on August 6, 2019 from, https://www.charlestonchronicle.net/2019/07/16/breast-cancer-is-the-most-imperative-health-issue-facing-african-american-women.

5 Vanderbilt University Medical Center. "Different subtypes of triple-negative breast cancer respond to different therapies." *ScienceDaily*. 27 June 2011. (www.sciencedaily.com/releases/2011/06/110627184000.htm).

6 Greenup R, Buchanan A, Lorizio W, Rhoads K, Chan S, Leedom T, et al. Prevalence of BRCA mutations among women with triple-negative breast cancer (TNBC) in a genetic counseling cohort. *Ann Surg Oncol*. 2013;20:3254–8.

7 Yam C, Mani SA, Moulder SL, Targeting the Molecular Subtypes of Triple-negative breast cancer: Understanding the Diversity to Progress the Field, *The Oncologist*. 2017;22:1086–1093.

8 Lehmann BC, Bauer JA, Chen Xi, et al. Identification of human triple-negative breast cancer subtypes and preclinical models for selection of targeted therapies, *J Clin Invest*. 2011;121(7):2750-2767. https://doi.org/10.1172/JCI45014.

9 *Breast Cancer Landscape*. Department of Defense Breast Cancer Research Program, 2019. Accessed on August 4, 2019 from, https://cdmrp.army.mil/bcrp/pdfs/bc_landscape.pdf.

10 Saraiva DP,Guadalupe Cabral M, Jacinto A, et al. How many diseases is triple neg-ative breast cancer: the protagonism of the immune microenvironment. ESMO Open 2017;2:e000208. doi:10.1136/ esmoopen-2017-000208.

11 Astvatsaturyan K, Yue Y, Walts AE, Bose S (2018). Androgen receptor positive triple-negative breast cancer: Clinicopathologic, prognostic, and predictive features. *PLoS ONE* 13(6): e0197827. https://doi.org/10.1371/journal.pone.0197827.

12 Lehmann BC, Bauer JA, Chen Xi, et al. Identification of human triple-negative breast cancer subtypes and preclinical models for selection of targeted therapies, *J Clin Invest*. 2011;121(7):2750-2767. https://doi.org/10.1172/JCI45014.

13 Astvatsaturyan K, Yue Y, Walts AE, Bose S (2018). Androgen receptor positive triple-negative breast cancer: Clinicopathologic, prognostic, and predictive features. PLoS ONE 13(6): e0197827. https://doi.org/10.1371/journal.pone.0197827.

14 Abramson VG, Lehmann BD, Ballinger TJ, et al. Subtyping of Triple-Negative Breast Cancer: Implications for Therapy. *Cancer*. 2014;121:8-16. VC 2014 Ameri-can Cancer Society.

15 Rampurwala M, Wisinski KB, O'Regan R, et. al. The Role of Androgen Receptor in Triple-Negative Breast Cancer. *Clin Adv Hematol Oncol*. 2016 March; 14(3): 186–193.

16 Sporikova Z, Koudelakova V, Trojanec R, et al. Genetic Markers in Triple-Negative Breast Cancer, *Clinical Breast Cancer*, Vol. 18, No. 5, e841-50 2018.

17 Broderick J, PARP Inhibitor Olaparib Outperforms Chemotherapy in BRCA-Posi-tive Breast Cancer, Accessed on June 19 from, https://www.oncnursingnews.com/printer?url=/web-exclusives/parp-inhibitor-ola-parib-outperforms-chemotherapy-in-brca-positive-breast-cancer.

18 Robson ME, Tung N, Conte P, et,al. OlympiAD final overall survival and tolerabil-ity results: Olaparib versus chemotherapy treatment of physician's choice in pa-tients with a germline BRCA mutation and HER2-negative metastatic breast cancer, *Annals of Oncology* 30: 558–566, 2019 doi:10.1093/annonc/mdz012 Published on-line 23 January 2019.

19 ttps://www.tnbcfoundation.org/research/medical-conference-updates/san-antonio-breast-cancer-symposium, 2018.

20 Thomas K, Ornstein C, Memorial Sloan Kettering's Chief Executive Resigns from Merck's Board of Directors, *The New York Times*, retrieved on June 1, 2019 from: https://www.nytimes.com/2018/10/02/health/memorial-sloan-kettering-thompson-merck.html.

21 Kim C, Gao R, Chemoresistance Evolution in Triple-Negative Breast Cancer Delin-eated by Single-Cell Sequencing, *Cell*. 2018 May 3;173(4):879-893.e13. doi: 10.1016/j.cell.2018.03.041. Epub 2018 Apr 19.

22 Carter D, *ARTEMIS clinical trial offers triple-negative patients personalized ther-apy*, accessed on June 3, 2019 from, https://www.mdanderson.org/publications/can-cer-frontline/breast-cance...090.html?Cmpid=twitter_frontline_TNBC_breast_moonshots_clinicaltrials.

23 MDAnderson.org, accessed on June 3, 2019 from, https://www.mdanderson.org/patients-family/diagnosis-treatment/clinical-trials/clinical-trials-index/clinical-trials-detail.ID2014-0185.html.

Chapter 9: Appendix

1 Lehmann BC, Bauer JA, Chen Xi, et al. Identification of human triple-negative breast cancer subtypes and preclinical models for selection of targeted therapies, J Clin Invest. 2011;121(7):2750-2767. https://doi.org/10.1172/JCI45014.

2 Xi Chen, Jiang Li, William H., TNBCtype: A Subtyping Tool for Triple-Negative Breast Cancer, *Cancer Informatics*.

3 Masuda H, Baggerly KA, Wang Y, et al. Differential response to neoadjuvant chemotherapy among 7 triple-negative breast cancer molecular subtypes. *Clin Cancer Res*. 2013 Oct 1;19(19):5533-40. doi: 10.1158/1078-0432.CCR-13-0799.

4 Yu KD, Zhu R, Zhan M, et al. Identification of prognosis-relevant subgroups in patients with chemoresistant triple-negative breast cancer. Clin Cancer Res. 2013; 19(10):2723–2733.

5 Santonja A, Albanell J, Chacon JI, et al. Triple-negative breast cancer subtypes and pathologic complete-response rate to neoadjuvant chemotherapy: Results from the GEICAM/2006-2003 study. *Journal of Clinical Oncology* 2014 32:15_suppl, 1024-1024.

6 Abramson VG, Lehmann BD, Ballinger TJ, et al. Subtyping of Triple-Negative Breast Cancer: Implications for Therapy. *Cancer*. 2014;121:8-16.

7 Rampurwala M, Wisinski KB, O'Regan R, et. al. The Role of Androgen Receptor in Triple-Negative Breast Cancer. *Clin Adv Hematol Oncol*. 2016 March; 14(3): 186–193.

8 Jézéquel P, Loussouarn D, Catherine Guérin-Charbonnel C, et. al. Gene-expression molecular subtyping of triple-negative breast cancer tumours: importance of immune response, *Breast Cancer Research* (2015).

9 Lehmann BD, Jovanović B, Chen X, Estrada MV, Johnson KN, Shyr Y, et al. (2016) Refinement of Triple-Negative Breast Cancer Molecular Subtypes: Implications for Neoadjuvant Chemotherapy Selection. *PLoS ONE* 11(6): e0157368. doi:10.1371/journal.pone.0157368.

10 Marotti JD, B. de Abreu F, Wells WA, et al. Triple-Negative Breast Cancer Next-Generation Sequencing for Target Identification. *The American Journal of Pathology*, Vol. 187, No. 10, October 2017.

11 Sporikova Z, Koudelakova V, Trojanec R, et. al. Genetic Markers in Triple-Negative Breast Cancer, *Clinical Breast Cancer*, Vol. 18, No. 5, e841-50.

Epilogue

1 Saraiva DP,Guadalupe Cabral M, Jacinto A, et al. How many diseases is triple negative breast cancer: the protagonism of the immune microenvironment. ESMO Open 2017;2:e000208. doi:10.1136/ esmoopen-2017-000208.

2 Cancer.gov, accessed on July 16, 2019 from, https://www.cancer.gov/publications/dictionaries/cancer-terms/def/tumor-infiltrating-lymphocyte.

3 Althobiti M, Aleskandarany MA, Joseph C, et al, Heterogeneity of tumour-infiltrating lymphocytes in breast cancer and its prognostic significance, *Histopathology*. 2018 Dec;73(6):887-896. doi: 10.1111/his.13695. Epub 2018 Oct 9.

4 Anders CK, Zagar TM, and Carey LA, Department of Medicine, Division of Hematology, University of North Carolina at Chapel Hill, Lineberger Comprehensive Cancer Center, *Hematol Oncol Clin North Am*. 2013 August ; 27(4): 737–749. doi:10.1016/j.hoc.2013.05.003.

5 Carey LA, Directed Therapy of Subtypes of Triple-Negative Breast Cancer, *The Oncologist* 2011;16(suppl 1):71–78. Retrieved from: www.TheOncologist.com.

6 Stewart RL, Updike KL, Factor RE, et al. A multigene assay determines risk of recurrence in patients with triple-negative breast cancer, 2019 *American Association for Cancer Research*, Retrieved from: cancerres.aacrjournals.org on June 17, 2019.

7 Hopkinsmedicine.org, accessed on July 16, 2019 from, (https://www.hopkinsmedicine.org/kimmel_cancer_center/research_clinical_trials/clinical_trials/mistletoe.html).

8 Cancer.gov, accessed on July 16, 2019 from, https://www.cancer.gov/about-cancer/treatment/cam/hp/mistletoe-pdq.